THE LEAN MACHINES

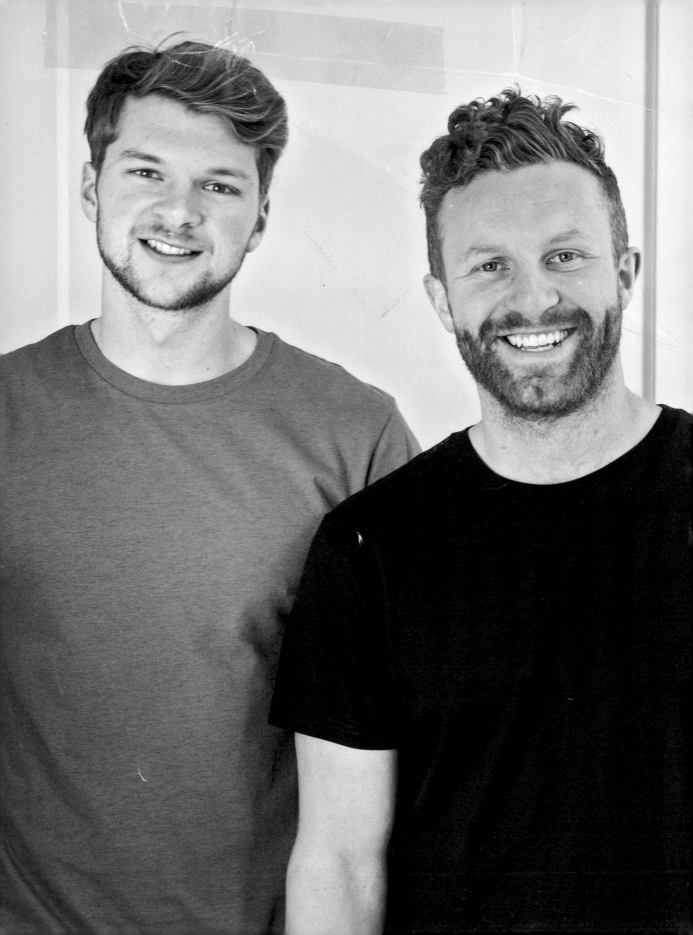

THE LEAN MACHINES

EAT WELL, MOVE BETTER & FEEL AWESOME

JOHN CHAPMAN and LEON BUSTIN

headline

First published in 2016
by HEADLINE PUBLISHING GROUP

1

Cataloguing in Publication Data is available from the British Library

Trade Paperback ISBN 978 1 4722 3626 5

Designed by Well Made Studio
Photography © Laurie Fletcher
Recipe development and food styling by Rich Harris
Edited by Laura Herring
Props styling by Jemima Hetherington

Printed and bound in Italy by L.E.G.O. S.p.A

Headline's policy is to use papers that are natural, renewable and recyclable products and made
from wood grown in sustainable forests. The logging and manufacturing processes are expected to
conform to the environmental regulations of the country of origin.

This book and the advice it contains is based on our personal experiences of working towards
becoming awesome mentally and physically. We are not qualified to give mental health advice,
and while our mindfulness tools work for us, they are not a substitute for professional advice.
Before following any diet or workout plan you should consult a doctor - what works for us as
personal trainers may not be suitable for everyone reading this book. If you are not used to
working out, before starting a new fitness routine you should: a) seek medical advice if needed
before starting, b) take things at a steady pace and remember not to do advanced exercises
until you are ready, c) stop all exercise and consult a doctor if you feel at all unwell. If you are
under sixteen you should consult your parents before making any changes to your diet, exercise
routine or lifestyle. And please look after yourself!

HEADLINE PUBLISHING GROUP
An Hachette UK Company
Carmelite House
50 Victoria Embankment
London EC4 0DZ

www.headline.co.uk
www.hachette.co.uk

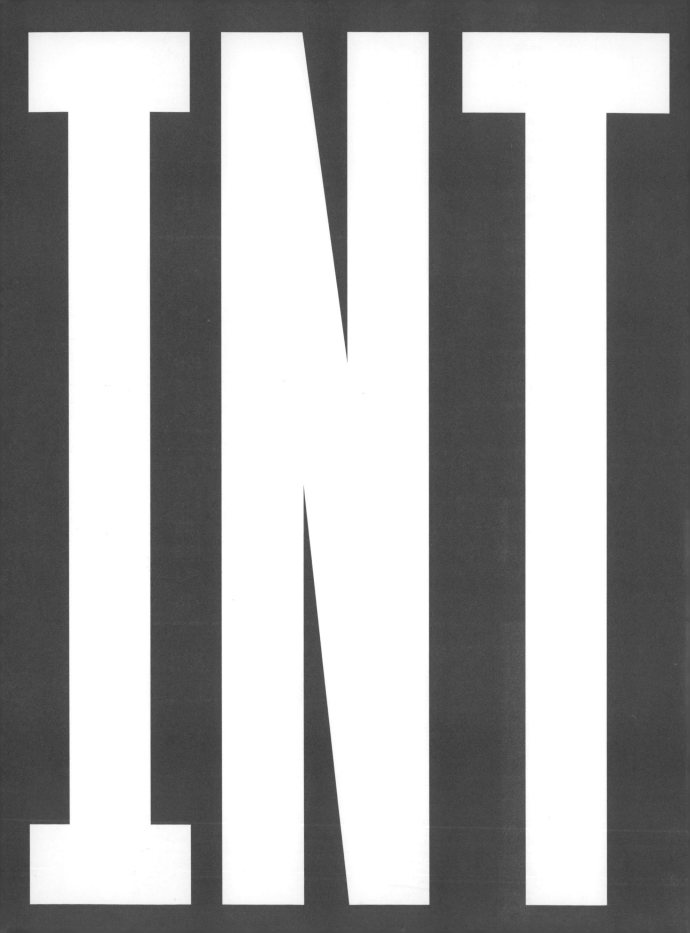

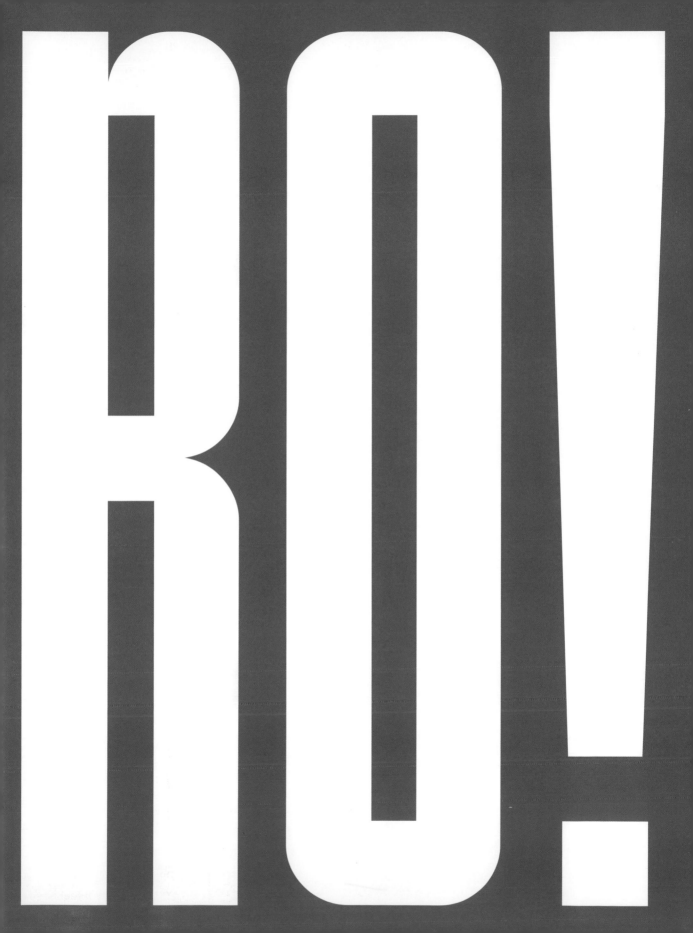

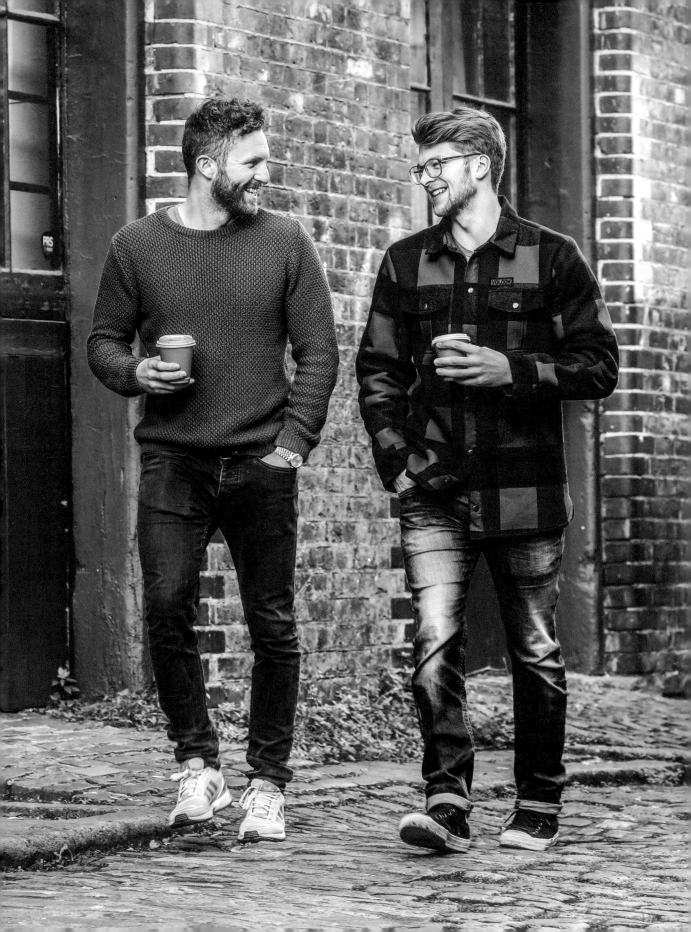

PROJECT AWESOME

YOUR GUIDE TO HEALTH AND HAPPINESS

We are The Lean Machines, otherwise known as Leon Bustin and John Chapman, and we're tired of seeing so many unhappy people around. Whether it's work, your lifestyle, your health or how you think you look that's bringing you down – or maybe it's more of a general feeling of being a little bit lost – we've created this book to make you aware of just how **awesome** you already are. And over the coming pages we'll share all the happiness, nutrition and fitness tools that we use every day so that you can become even more awesome!

We're best mates and health coaches who are passionate about making the world a healthier and happier place. Over our years in the fitness and so-called 'health industry' we've worked with people from all walks of life and at all stages of their fitness goals. We know that a worrying number of us feel insecure about our bodies – and we also know that the media doesn't help. With 'perfect' Photoshopped bodies on the covers of magazines and billboards, it can be hard to have confidence in ourselves, but we're here to tell you that

everyone has a right to be happy and to feel good about themselves. In the chapters that follow we will show you how.

We don't really support quick detoxes, fad diets or claims of 'Drop a Dress Size in Two Weeks'. We're all about small changes that you can keep up long term. Yes, you will probably lose a lot of weight in ten days if all you are eating is smoothies, but in our experience all that weight – and often more – will go straight back on again and you will quickly revert to your old habits. It's just not sustainable – physically or mentally – to live this way, not to mention that the weight you will lose is likely to be not only fat but also muscle that we desperately need to hold on to. We also want to draw attention away from such a keen focus on how much we weigh. Feeling awesome is about so much more than this. It's about being healthy and active, and taking proper time to look after your mind as well as your body. That's why we start the book with a whole chapter on being happy!

We think it is *that* important.

We really want to teach you something that you won't struggle to maintain – a few lifestyle changes that will keep you in shape without sacrificing your happiness at the same time. Getting fit and healthy should be fun! Of course, if you need to lose fat, then there will be some sacrifices to make, such as eating less, but if you understand why you're doing it and how amazing you'll feel when you're fitter and healthier, we think you'll enjoy the process so much more and you'll be able to keep going.

On leaving school we both went into trade jobs – as a roof tiler and a carpenter. We owe so much to and have so much respect for the people we met while doing that hugely physically demanding work, but we knew that we couldn't see ourselves climbing around on roofs on cold winter days into our fifties and sixties. But more than that, we knew we were destined to work in the fitness industry. What we really wanted to do was to help people take a leap of faith into the unknown and to be a part of their positive process on the way to changing their lives. We wanted to help people overcome their fears. When the recession hit, the building industry ground to a halt but, bizarrely, for us it was actually a good thing – looking back, the best thing that could have happened really. When the boss's phone stopped ringing and work became thin on the ground, we were forced to make a decision to do something else. It was either that or wait it out, which wasn't an option…

We pulled together as much money as we could and got qualified as fitness instructors. And then we went travelling so we could see some of the world. On our separate adventures we met the most amazing and wonderful people, full of passion and a real zest for life. It was definitely our wake-up call. On returning to the UK, Leon hassled the manager of his local gym (Shaun, who is now a really good friend!) until he gave him a job…as a receptionist! And John carried on as a carpenter for another few months while continuing his studies in his spare time. In the following years we worked our butts off and we haven't slowed down since. As a result, we've gone from being employed by a gym to running our own businesses in a pretty short space of time.

We are constantly looking to learn more through working with our clients both in and out of the gym, listening to podcasts, reading piles of books, speaking to friends and attending seminars by the best in the industry. Amazingly, as a result of putting ourselves out there, we were actually lucky enough to become very good friends with a few of those same people we looked up to when we were starting out and still admire so much today! It's so true that you get out what you put in. Yes, we work long hours, yes we get up very early – but we love it! We feel so lucky that we can say, hand on heart, that we love our job.

Fast forward to right now and here we are, aged twenty-eight, sitting in a coffee shop sharing our message and experiences with you. It's so surreal to look back and realise that everything that has happened to us came from what most people would call a negative situation: losing our jobs. Shifting your mindset, looking for opportunities and taking a jump into the unknown can make all the difference to achieving happiness and your goals (more of that later!).

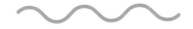

ANYWAY, ENOUGH ABOUT US! THIS BOOK IS ALL ABOUT

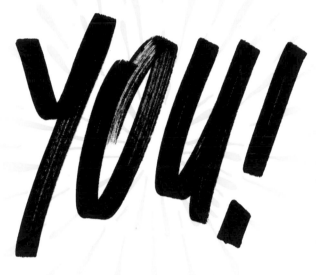

First things first: this book is for everyone who is on a journey towards health, fitness and finding balance in everything you do. Whether you're already on your way and need a bit of a steer in the right direction, or you're just thinking about getting started and are not sure which way to turn, see this book as your 'complete guide to health and happiness'! This is NOT your ordinary, generic fitness book claiming to get you jacked and ripped or suggesting that you eat nothing but dust for the next eight weeks to get a bikini body. We will cut through all the advice out there – from the TV to the latest fads to what you heard from your mate down the gym – and let you know what is real, what is achievable and how you can reach those goals. We want to cut straight to the simple facts that are proven to work. No false claims.

Our belief is that good health is a lot more than a perfectly balanced meal or a chiseled six-pack; it's also – and most importantly – about YOU. In the western world most of us have the wealth and lifestyles others can only dream about, but sadly many of us are still looking for the magic ingredient to make our lives somehow better. We have all the technology we need to make our lives easier, but we're more stressed than ever before. Often we think that if we get that dream job or promotion or pay rise, or a bigger house, we will be happy. And often we *are* happier – for a little while at least – but it's not long before we're thinking about the next thing on our list.

Something we come back to often is a study conducted into happiness that was published in *The Journal of Personality and Social Psychology**. It compared the happiness of individuals who had just won the lottery with those who had just experienced accidents resulting in paralysis. Unsurprisingly, the lottery winners had a huge initial peak in happiness while the others naturally experienced a big drop in happiness. But what's interesting is that pretty soon afterwards, both returned to their normal basal happiness levels. The highs and lows of life are inevitable but usually temporary. Our bodies, our life, our friends and our partners will all change over the years, our wealth will go up and down, our health may suffer, but to be truly happy we need to accept and work with this fact. We could all do with spending more time looking for the good in life, and learning from the negatives. It's time we stopped looking at the external world for happiness and instead started looking inside. We want to show you the tools that work for us!

*Lottery winners and accident victims: is happiness relative?, Brickman P, Coates D, Janoff-Bulman R. *Journal of Personality and Social Psychology*, 1978, Vol. 36, No. 8, 917–927

HOW AWESOME DO YOU FEEL?

Rate your answers between 1 and 5 on our scale of awesomeness
(where 5 is positively awesome and 1 is not very awesome at all).

BE HAPPY

Are you happy? _____

What kinds of things do you do to relax? _____
_____

How much do you love yourself?   ① ② ③ ④ ⑤
How stressed do you feel?   ① ② ③ ④ ⑤
What makes you feel scared, anxious, worried or unhappy? _____
_____

Would you say you have a generally positive outlook on life? ① ② ③ ④ ⑤

NUTRITION

How healthy would you say your diet is?   ① ② ③ ④ ⑤

How many meals each week do you cook from scratch? _____

How much water do you drink per day? _____

How much do you enjoy cooking?   ① ② ③ ④ ⑤

Do you feel you have enough energy?   ① ② ③ ④ ⑤

FITNESS

On average how many hours of unbroken sleep do you get each night? _____

How many times do you exercise a week?*   ① ② ③ ④ ⑤+
*we mean getting sweaty for at least 20 minutes

What are your top 3 fitness goals?   1. _____
                                       2. _____
                                       3. _____

How much do you enjoy exercise?   ① ② ③ ④ ⑤

How happy are you with your body?   ① ② ③ ④ ⑤

SETTING THE RIGHT GOALS

So, before we dive into the juicy bits of this book, let's take a few minutes to find out a bit more about you and what makes you tick. We've put together the questionnaire opposite so that you can identify the areas of your life that could do with a bit of The Lean Machines love. Then use your answers to these questions to set some truly achievable goals, using the advice and guidance in the rest of the book.

MOTIVATION IS WHAT GETS YOU STARTED, HABIT IS WHAT KEEPS YOU GOING.

JIM RYAN

Looking at the answers you gave, did you score yourself less than three on any of them? Were any of your answers difficult to write down? These are the first areas that we should focus on. The following chapters all contain easy-to-use, practical advice and great information to help you achieve all of your happiness, nutrition and fitness goals. However, it's important to set yourself some achievable, workable goals; it's a good idea to start off with some easy ones, like making sure you drink enough water each day. Others may need a bit of work, such as enjoying cooking more (our delicious recipes will soon convince you it's worth it though!) and increasing the amount that you exercise each week.

You'll quickly find that most of the areas above are closely interlinked. Once you start making a positive change in one part of your life, the others will quickly follow. When you find an exercise routine that you enjoy, you'll do it more often, and if you do it more often then your

body will quickly start to look and feel better. As you feel better physically, your self worth will improve, and as your self worth improves, so will your confidence to try new exercises and foods. As what you eat improves, so will your general health, appearance and quality of sleep, and as your sleep improves, your stress levels and recovery will get better, which will all help improve your overall happiness. It's all part of one continuous journey.

Change just one thing for the better: address the most urgent aspect of your lifestyle and the others will all start to come into line too! Maybe you want to start with cooking a few meals from scratch each week? We promise that if you do that, you'll instantly have more of an awareness of what you're putting into your body, and it will make you more conscious of your other actions – you'll then start to make better choices elsewhere in your life.

Now, on to the book!

HOW THIS BOOK WORKS

The book is split into three parts, each focussing on the most important aspects of happiness, nutrition and fitness. Although they are separate, they are carefully designed to work together, to help you on your way to total health and happiness.

The truth is, getting into great shape doesn't have to be so hard if you concentrate your efforts in the right areas, setting a few clear goals, rather than spreading yourself across lots of areas. It's all about efficiency. The most common issue we come across in the gym is that people want to achieve everything all at once, or they are looking for an easy, quick fix. We often see people wondering what supplement they should take next, when really their diet sucks and they should start there first. It's the same in all areas of your well-being – start small and look at the bigger picture.

PART 1: BE HAPPY

- In this section we will show the importance of positive thinking and teach you how to take better control of your thoughts and banish negativity.
- We will arm you with our eight top tools for bringing more happiness to your everyday life and show you our practical exercises for building confidence and reducing stress.
- We share our personal experiences and help you to set achievable goals for a life with more happiness and positivity.

PART 2: EAT WELL

- We will help you work out what your ideal daily calorie intake should be based on your activity levels – the most important factor in losing fat or building muscle.
- We will provide you with a deeper understanding of what macronutrients are (the fats, carbohydrates and proteins in your food), where they come from and how much of each you need every day.
- Enjoy 60 awesome recipes all with calorie and macronutrient breakdowns, to get you creating amazing, tasty food while keeping you on track.

PART 3: MOVE BETTER

- We will show you why exercise is so important and exactly where to focus your efforts to get the best results.
- Step-by-step photos show you how to safely perform our key exercises, along with top tips and hints for maximum impact.
- We provide individualised training plans suitable for all fitness levels and goals, for the gym and at home, plus HIIT (High Intensity Interval Training) sessions and circuits.

LET'S MAKE THIS OFFICIAL!

I PROMISE THAT I WILL:

①

Create 3–5 affirmations to repeat throughout my day. These will reinforce my new, positive thinking patterns. (See pages 24–25.)

②

Become more aware of my thoughts and feelings and not let external events dictate my happiness.

③

I will obey the 80/20 rule: 80 per cent of the time I will eat healthy single ingredient foods, knowing that as long as I stick to my calories I can still enjoy some balance in life.

④

I will complete my food diary for 1 week, as instructed on page 50.

⑤

I will exercise 3–5 times a week for at least 30 minutes.

⑥

I will learn to understand happiness is not the final destination, but a way I choose to live.

SIGNED: _____   DATE: _____

WITNESS: _____

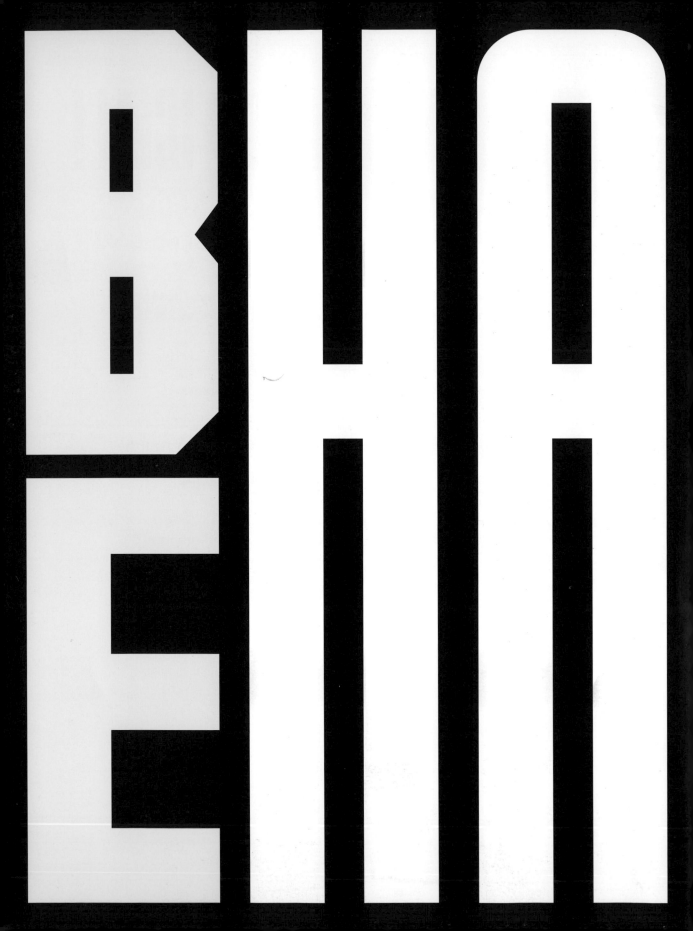

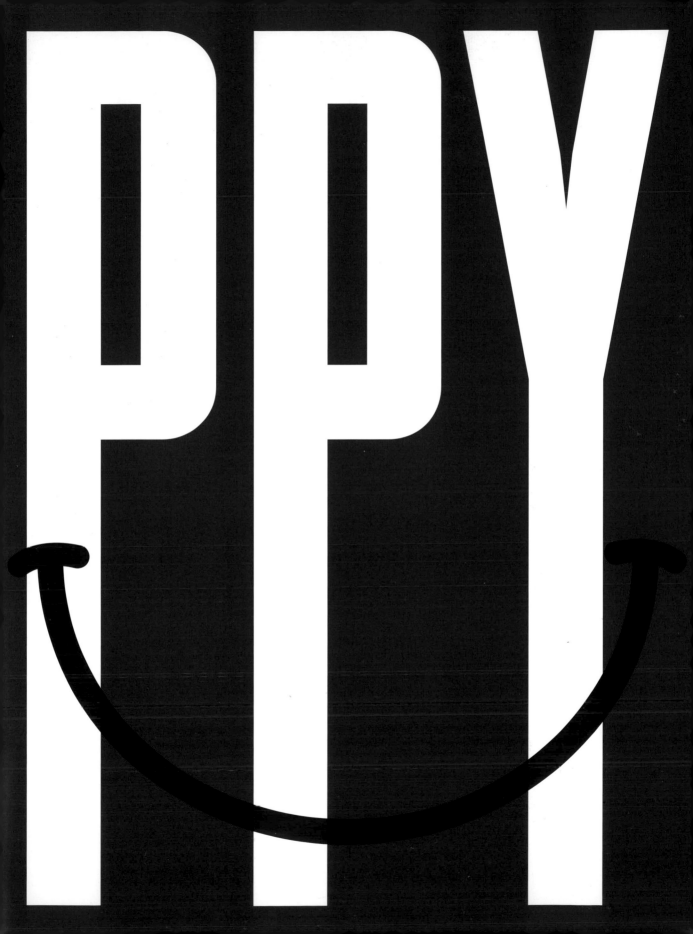

WHAT IS *HAPPINESS?*

IN THIS SECTION WE WILL SHOW THE IMPORTANCE OF POSITIVE THINKING AND TEACH YOU HOW TO TAKE BETTER CONTROL OF YOUR THOUGHTS AND BANISH NEGATIVITY.

WE WILL ARM YOU WITH OUR EIGHT TOP TOOLS FOR BRINGING MORE HAPPINESS TO YOUR EVERYDAY LIFE AND SHOW YOU OUR PRACTICAL EXERCISES FOR BUILDING CONFIDENCE AND REDUCING STRESS.

WE SHARE OUR PERSONAL EXPERIENCES AND HELP YOU TO SET ACHIEVABLE GOALS FOR A LIFE WITH MORE HAPPINESS AND POSITIVITY.

First things first. Although we want you to look and feel great, we all need to understand that a six-pack, twenty-inch guns or a perfectly round butt will not bring you happiness, contrary to what the magazine covers claim. They may raise your confidence and give you a temporary, much-needed boost, but they will not sustain your happiness long term. In some cases, a 'perfect' body can even become a negative tie, as getting into great shape is often followed by the pressure to stay looking that way. Always remember that you are more than just your physical appearance.

Over the following pages, we will reveal our top tips and practical activities for introducing more happiness into your life. We will help you identify who you really are and what you want from life, helping you to include more of what makes you happy and eliminate those behaviours that have a negative impact on your happiness. By the end of this chapter you will be feeling more confident, happy and in control.

But before we get started, let us ask you a simple YES or NO question:

Are you happy?

Now, we bet most people reading this thought something like this:

What, right now?
Yes.
Of course I am
Aren't I?
Am I?
Well sometimes I am,
or at least I will be when...

If you answered like that you are probably not living in the present! And if you are not living in the present you will never be truly happy, as the past has been and the future is never promised.

We will let John explain...

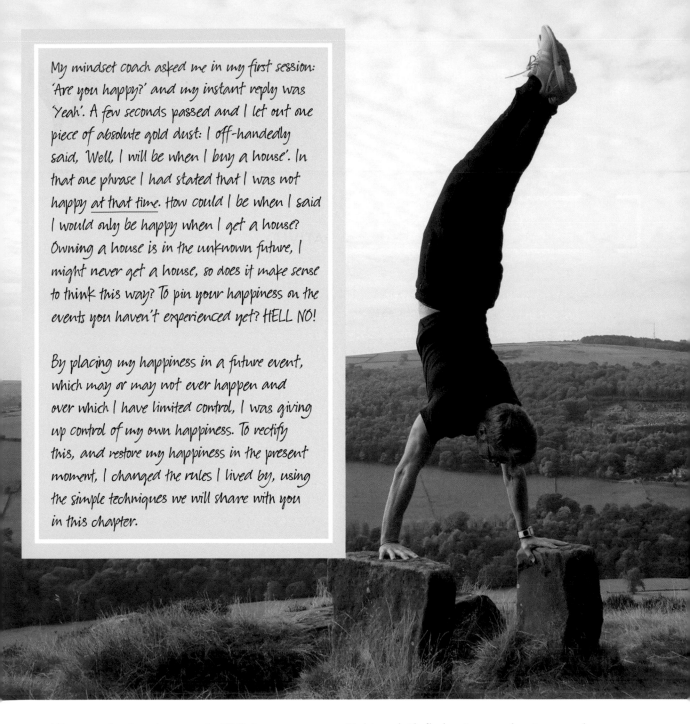

My mindset coach asked me in my first session: 'Are you happy?' and my instant reply was 'Yeah'. A few seconds passed and I let out one piece of absolute gold dust: I off-handedly said, 'Well, I will be when I buy a house'. In that one phrase I had stated that I was not happy at that time. How could I be when I said I would only be happy when I get a house? Owning a house is in the unknown future, I might never get a house, so does it make sense to think this way? To pin your happiness on the events you haven't experienced yet? HELL NO!

By placing my happiness in a future event, which may or may not ever happen and over which I have limited control, I was giving up control of my own happiness. To rectify this, and restore my happiness in the present moment, I changed the rules I lived by, using the simple techniques we will share with you in this chapter.

We are going to set you up to WIN, because let's be honest, every day that you wake up in the morning and your heart is still pumping is a GOOD day.

Right, so let's find out more about you and what makes you happy and work on getting more happiness into your everyday life.

WHO ARE YOU?

> **'YOU ARE THE MASTER OF YOUR OWN DESTINY...
> BELIEVE IT, IT'S TRUE.'** NAPOLEON HILL

This might seem like some sort of cryptic question, but in order for any of us to make real long-term changes and to find balance in body and mind, we must first look at ourselves and ask the questions of who and what we really are right now. Through the answers we can then pave the way to becoming the version of ourselves we ultimately would like to be.

Working with our clients, we have come across so many wonderful people who held no value in the person they were, placing all of their happiness in the future, whether it be an event, their physique, job, salary – or even becoming a parent. This absolutely crushes us, but we get it, we were those people too.

We are all sold on the idea that when we get to the next level, that's when we will be truly happy. But often when we reach those goals, instead of enjoying them, we are worried about keeping that new job, or whether we even deserved it in the first place! So many of us live in fear of what hasn't even happened yet, and this is hugely damaging to our happiness.

Quite simply what we're trying to say is that, yes, it is fantastic (and important) to have goals to work towards, in the short, mid and long term – in fact, we think they're vital

(see pages 22–23) – but in order to find true happiness and balance, we must first find happiness in the present moment. We can't go back and we sure as hell can't fast-forward, so we might as well enjoy the ride.

As well as pinning happiness on future events, lots of people try to live in the past – either reliving a time when they felt more confident, were fitter or had more money, or carrying around regret or guilt about something they did or didn't do. Past events are definitely worth talking to a professional about if they are affecting your day-to-day life. But we think that we can also use our past experiences to help shape our present: if you are upset about the way you behaved in the past, use this to positively influence how you behave today.

The sad thing is it's often only when a truly life-changing event happens – such as facing illness or losing a loved one – that we gain clarity about what's really important to us in life, and subsequently let go of our petty fears. All that really matters in life are the bonds we make and the love we share. Do you think on your deathbed you will be thinking about all the money you made or how big your house is? I think we all know the answer to that one.

So let's answer a few more questions to find out more about you. It's really important that you answer all of these questions one-hundred per cent honestly, as they will help you work out what means the most to you and which areas could do with a bit of improvement.

DO YOU ENJOY YOUR JOB? _____

WHAT DO YOU DO FOR FUN? _____

HOW MANY HOURS A WEEK DO YOU GET TO DO WHAT YOU REALLY ENJOY? _____

WHAT MAKES YOU SAD? _____

HOW CONFIDENT DO YOU FEEL? _____

WOULD YOU SAY YOU'RE A WORRIER? _____

DO YOU THINK YOU'RE LIVING TO YOUR FULL POTENTIAL? _____

WHO ARE YOUR BEST FRIENDS? _____

ARE THOSE FRIENDS SUPPORTIVE? _____

WHAT DOES WEALTH MEAN TO YOU? _____

DO YOU FEEL UNDER PRESSURE TO LOOK A CERTAIN WAY? _____

WHAT BRINGS YOU THE MOST HAPPINESS IN YOUR LIFE? _____

IS THERE ANYTHING THAT YOU FEEL IS HOLDING YOU BACK? _____

Take a look at your answers. Did any of them make you smile? Were any particularly painful to think about? There are probably some areas that you know immediately you should spend a bit of time thinking about and working on. What did you write for the question 'What do you do for fun?' Was it an easy one to think about, or did it make you realise you could do with more fun in your daily routine? The last question is a big one. Really think about it, and make a note of any feelings surrounding your answer. Nothing should be holding you back!

SETTING ACHIEVABLE *GOALS*

What is an achievable goal?, we hear you ask.

First it's set with one thing in mind: you! There's no point setting goals that you think your partner or friends will think are awesome. Setting a goal for yourself will mean you instantly invest more of yourself into it.

Secondly, set a goal over which you have control of the outcome. For instance, setting a goal of 'I want to be able to run 5k with Jason every Wednesday' is a great goal (in that a 5k run would be awesome), but you are not in control of Jason (whoever Jason is) and if he decides at 3k that he's had enough and is going to the pub, then it's going to be harder for you to motivate yourself beyond that point.

Thirdly, set yourself up to win! Set goals that, yes, will test you and mean you have to work hard to achieve them, but don't set them either so far in the future that you'll never get there or so hard that you're going to have to sacrifice too much of your happiness to even get close. Don't get us wrong, to get in great shape you will have to make sacrifices, but we don't see why your happiness should be one of them.

Finally, break it down into smaller goals. As humans, we are results-driven; we like to win, or at least feel like we are. So setting goals with this in mind will help us stay motivated in the long term. Think of your end goal, but then break it down into little goals along the way, so you can celebrate each one when you reach it.

This process of setting both short- and long-term goals will also teach you to stop and assess your position along the way. It's very easy to get wrapped up in a goal we wanted at day one and blindly become a slave to it. But as we evolve and change, so too can our goals. Having the confidence to actually listen to yourself, to your body and what you really want is key.

That's why, in our opinion, those 'six-week SHRED' or 'twelve weeks OF HELL' plans don't really work. Well, we'll rephrase that; we don't believe they work long term. Most of these plans are set up with one thing in mind: your transformation photo being shared so the company can sell more plans. Sure, you will drop weight and or body fat (if that's the goal), but what these plans breed is a short-term attitude. Most people we work with want their dream body in next-to-no time and honestly don't really care too much how they get there – they just want it NOW. But the big question we need to ask ourselves is, what next?

Let's use an example from Leon's past to show how setting goals and breaking them down into smaller steps can make them less daunting and more manageable:

I decided that I really wanted to go travelling to see Australia, New Zealand and Thailand. I planned to allow two years before getting on that plane to give me time save up enough money. I worked out that the ticket, plus spending money added up to £8,000 – WHAAAAAAT?! Reaching that number was my long-term goal.

Once I had set that goal, which seemed a huge mountain to climb, I tracked back to decide a plan of action in order for me to achieve it – and to get me on that plane! I started by saying, 'Right, I'm going to save the same amount each month until I go', meaning that for 24 months I had to save £333.30 every single month. Each month would see me a step closer, achieving a comparatively small goal that over time would add up to a HUGE achievement (or amount of money).

This is a very simple example of breaking down what may seem, on the face of it, to be a huge goal. Chopping it into smaller chunks and ticking them off as you go makes it a lot more manageable and you can really chart your success. But, of course, the plan only works in an ideal world; goals and journeys are not a simple, linear process. I had bumps in the road: months where I didn't save enough – but then there were some months when I'd manage to save more. Whatever happened though, I always kept one eye on that long-term goal.

It may not always be easy or go to plan, and sometimes you will have to adapt in order to make that end goal happen, but by keeping it in sight and putting every ember of your being into the right here and now, constantly moving towards it, you will get there.

We want every single person we meet to be committed to themselves, their body and their health for the rest of their lives. So if you want to get shredded for a holiday in the space of 6 weeks, then that's fine, but our stance is this:

be more-or-less where you want to be, both physically and mentally, all year round, instead of becoming a slave to the gym for six weeks of the year. It's important to achieve balance in life (more of this on page 33), that way you can spend more time thinking about what you're actually going to do on your holiday instead.

Now, let's look at our eight tools of happiness to help you achieve your goals and generally feel more positive every single day.

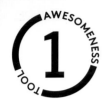

AWARENESS
AND CREATING YOUR OWN POSITIVE AFFIRMATIONS

Awareness is absolutely essential in order to achieve happiness.

You can achieve awareness by asking yourself questions or simply by sitting and looking inwards. You'll probably find that sometimes it can be a bit uncomfortable digging into how you are really feeling deep down. But it's so important that you do, in order to be true to yourself and to grow as a person. So, next time you feel down, or someone says something in conversation and for some reason it makes you feel unhappy, remember it. And then when you can, think back to it and ask yourself why it bothered you. Why? Why? Why? Do this until you find a root cause. Then ask yourself if it makes sense and is reasonable.

Most of the beliefs that we use and rely on every day were instilled in us long before we reached adulthood. People so often repeat what their friends have told them, or what their parents brought them up to believe, but often those opinions aren't beneficial to *you*. One size does not fit all! Once we identify those deep-rooted beliefs we can then begin to question them.

Once you identify a belief or thought pattern that is making you unhappy, we promise you have the power to change it. You are the only one who can choose and control your thoughts.

We all need to strip those outdated thoughts away and create a new set of affirmations to live by.

Affirmations are a set of phrases that you repeat daily to yourself with conviction until you adopt them as an innate part of you. Pick a regular time of day – or several times a day – to remind yourself of them. Say them out loud with conviction.

Thinking back to John's experience with his mindset coach on page 19, let's take a walk through what happened next.

After John's session, he went away and came up with a new positive affirmation:

··

I am in the peace of this present moment.

··

This helped John remain in the now, rather than uselessly worrying about the future. He repeated this ten times on his drive to work every day, in several convincing tones of voice, as though he were acting – and at first he was. When you're getting started, it can feel a bit silly talking to yourself out loud. But within a few weeks, you'll start to feel the powerful effects of positive affirmations. You won't just start believing what you say, you will start living it.

Make your first affirmation:

··

I am confident and I can do anything anyone else can do!

··

Maybe you feel disappointed that you don't get enough time each week to do the things you really love. Your new affirmation could be:

> **I will make time to do the things I enjoy because I deserve it.**

Or maybe you need to link your affirmations to specific situations in your daily life. Maybe your line manager at work scares the crap out of you! Make a new affirmation to repeat before your meetings:

> **I am confident in my abilities and I am good at my job.**

In our experience, affirmations are even more powerful if used while meditating. Meditation is a bit of a paradox because you are actively trying to think about nothing, but if you're trying to think about nothing, then you're thinking. See the conundrum here? How we learnt to start meditating was using a kneeling cushion and adopting a position with an upright spine and an ever-so-slightly tucked-in chin. We then place one hand on top of the other with palms facing up and thumbs touching. We then start to focus on our breathing while allowing ourselves to relax, we count to 10 using our breaths, and with each deep inhale and exhale we count 1, 2 and so on. The idea is to try and make it to 10 without letting your mind wander, by thinking about what's in tomorrow's workout plan, for example. This is very hard and to start with you may only be able to make it to 2, but as time progresses you will make it to 10, at which point you can start the count again.

It wasn't until we filmed with Jamie Oliver, a big idol of ours, that it really sank in how effective affirmations can be. John had a

moment where his affirmation popped into his head spontaneously and he instantly broke out into a huge smile, realising he really was living and breathing every moment of the experience. It sometimes happens that through being more aware of our own thoughts, we realise our negative feelings are actually nothing to do with any faulty belief patterns we may have, and there is actually another reason for them. John has a good example:

I'm normally ready to kick ass in the morning. Sure, the initial 5:30a.m. wake-up sucks, but I remind myself that I'm doing what I love, so I quickly changed my mindset and the morning becomes a lot easier. I start off by doing what Tom Cruise does in the film Jerry Maguire when he wakes up: he claps and says 'Today is gonna be a good day'. Give it a go tomorrow – it works! One particular morning I was driving to work and couldn't stop myself feeling negative, so I turned the radio off and asked myself why. I chased it back and the answer was alcohol! Alcohol makes me super-negative the day after drinking but I'd never noticed this before. When I was younger and used to drink on Saturday nights, I assumed that everyone got the Sunday blues, but for me it was more than that: alcohol is a very depressive substance for me. I sometimes still have a few drinks but I know what to expect the next day so I adjust for it and spend more time on myself.

Being aware means spending time looking inwards, thinking about why we react to situations in certain ways, how we feel day-to-day and identifying what can have a negative impact on our happiness. But it's also about acting on those discoveries. You are in control of your own happiness!

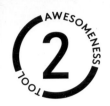

ACCEPTANCE

Sometimes things go wrong. They just don't work out as you had hoped, however much you thought they would. Maybe you lost your job, or a work project failed, or a relationship ended unexpectedly. When things don't go your way, you have a couple of options open to you. You can fight against it and struggle with all your might, or you can accept your situation and apply your efforts to working around the problem.

If you can learn to accept whatever life throws at you, then you will find you can cope with life's ups and down much more easily. Sure, you will still feel the pain of break-ups and losses, but if you can accept what has happened to you, you are halfway to successfully moving on.

Shakespeare has a great quote: 'Nothing is either good or bad, but thinking makes it so.' This is so true, as most things in life are not inherently bad or good and it just depends on the person's viewpoint. For example, do you remember in the first few pages where Leon explained how we had to leave our jobs or face losing them? To many people that would be a terrible situation, but to us it was an opportunity to progress, help others and find happiness. We accepted our situation and chose to work with it, rather than struggle against a situation we could not change: a declining economy. Again, this links to goal setting (see pages 22–23): we set ourselves up to win, rather than making a goal of being busy in a trade over which we had no control.

Honestly, how often does the worst actually happen? We like to think worst-case scenario but think back to the last time you had a crisis; do it now. Did the worst happen? Probably not, so maybe we should start looking more to the positive in situations and accept change with open arms. Think of it as swimming with the current instead of against it.

Sometimes we have to accept failure. This is often the hardest thing to do; but what if we change the way we see failure? What if we said to you:

'Failure is not a bad thing. If you're not failing you're not pushing yourself to your full potential.'

Now we're not expecting you to embrace this, nor are we setting you up to fail, but rather trying to show you how debilitating fear is and how to use the power of your thoughts to banish it. Just humour us and go with it: how much less scary would the world be if failure was perfectly normal and in fact commended when it came after trying hard?

After all, the only thing that is one-hundred per cent guaranteed in your life is CHANGE, and no, we don't mean that pocketful you have in the morning after a night out, but the fact that everything is and always will be changing. Learn to accept this and you will be making a monumental step towards reducing your stress and sky-rocketing your happiness.

CHANGE YOUR THOUGHTS AND YOU CHANGE YOUR WORLD

NORMAN VINCENT PEALE

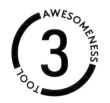

LOOK AFTER YOUR BODY

BODY IMAGE AND HAPPINESS

'LOOK AFTER YOUR BODY, IT'S THE ONLY PLACE YOU HAVE TO LIVE.'

JIM ROHN

Your body is beautiful and the only thing you will carry with you throughout your whole life, so it's only natural for it to change, adapt and move forward with you – it's already been through a lot! But looking after your body means so much more than looking good in a swimsuit. Being healthy and exercising properly has been proven to reduce stress and have a positive impact on so many other areas of your overall well-being. And once you feel like your body is on your side, you'll automatically feel more confident and full of energy to do all the other things you want to do. Who knew that going for a simple jog could be so good for you? But it's important to set the right goals.

Our world is obsessed with body image: what people look like and, more importantly (and scarily in our opinion), what people 'should' look like. We see client after client coming to us with fantastic bodies, relatively healthy and physically in a pretty damn good place to start with. But they all have one thing in common: they hate what they see staring back at them in the mirror. They sit and pick themselves apart bit by bit throughout the consultation process, to be left with maybe a left big toe and the dimples in their cheeks being the only things they actually like. Okay, so we're exaggerating here, but you know what we're trying to say!

When thinking about their body image goals, most people immediately refer to a celebrity or athlete they've seen on the cover of a magazine that they aspire to look like and throw around buzzwords like 'fit', 'muscly', 'skinny jeans'... We rarely hear the words 'healthy' and 'strong'. And very few of our clients initially set body goals with their own bodies in mind. It's like they are saying 'out with the old, in with the new'. But this doesn't really apply to our bodies. It's important to set healthy and realistic goals that you will stick to long term because training – however hard – isn't miraculously going to turn you into a totally new person. By no means is it our dream to banish all magazines from the world – far from it – but it's important to remember that not everyone wants the physique of a runner or body builder; nor should they feel pressure to look that way.

It becomes especially dangerous when people want to look a certain way so badly that they start doing things the unhealthy way or by spending loads of money. Almost every week we receive emails from new supplement companies promising that their brand will make all our dreams come true. All they are doing is playing to our insecurities and telling us what we want to hear. We get that everyone needs to make a living, and this industry will keep growing long after us, but what we want to make sure is that every single one of you reading this book is immune to all that nonsense.

Now let us guide you through how we set body image goals with our clients.

First, let's declutter and forget about the outside world for a minute. Imagine there are no celebrities with ripped torsos and no glossy magazines with bikini bods on the front. This is all about you and what you want. It is your journey, so let's find out what is important to you.

Ask yourself why you go to the gym. What do you want to achieve? What will actually make you happy? You'll probably find that it's not the major overhaul that you thought. You may even be thinking, 'is that it?' It's crazy how much external sources play a part on our goal-setting process. We only have to see one six-pack on a magazine and the panic sets in. Expectation grows, goals become more extreme, time becomes limited and, most of all, pressure builds up, leading to anxiety and often the fear to get started.

So what is your goal? Say it out loud. Maybe you want to lose a couple of kilos in weight and run 5k without stopping. From this point in, that's all you need to focus on: progressive weight loss and training to increase your ability to run 5k. Any research you do should be only about those two things (see our chapters on Nutrition and Fitness for more on these). And you don't need to achieve your goal overnight! Be kind to yourself; if you've a way to go to get to your goal, that's perfectly fine – and if it takes a bit longer, then all that means is that you're making your fitness goals a part of your longer-term lifestyle, which means they're more likely to stick. Sometimes if we achieve our goals too quickly, we can find ourselves on a slippery slope back to where we started.

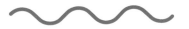

This is a classic technique for training and goal setting, based on the idea of decluttering – removing all external influences and expectations. And we can do this in all aspects of our life, from work and relationships to hobbies. The second we stop buying into the expectations thrust upon us, we suddenly start to shine and enjoy the ride a whole lot more. Why is this? Because we are riding our own wave, not anybody else's and it feels a lot more worthwhile mentally and physically. So remember, your body is as beautiful as YOU say it is.

Encourage yourself! Sometimes the only good things your hear about yourself will come from you, so be sure to shower yourself with positive affirmations and encouragement.

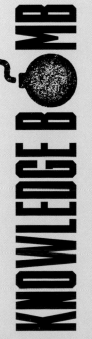

KNOWLEDGE BOMB

DID YOU KNOW IN AMERICA MOST SUPPLEMENTS ARE UNTESTED BY ANY EXTERNAL BODY AND IF THE FOOD AND DRUG ADMINISTRATION (FDA) WANTS TO REMOVE A SUPPLEMENT BECAUSE IT'S NOT DEEMED SAFE, THEY HAVE TO FIRST PROVE THAT IT'S NOT SAFE!

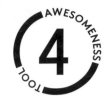

TACKLING THE BIG WORD... ANXIETY

Anxiety is a huge, HUGE subject and is a key area to cover when discussing happiness. There are so many misconceptions surrounding anxiety, and people often underestimate the devastating effect it can have on someone's life and training.

So first up, what is it? In the medical world anxiety is classified as a feeling of nervousness or worry over an uncertain outcome – feeling like you don't have control in a certain environment or over a situation. Breaking it down a bit further, there are two main types: 'specific-based anxiety', which means a sufferer has specific triggers that bring up those overwhelmingly anxious feelings, such as seeing spiders or being in big crowds. The other is 'generalised anxiety', which can have more of an impact on day-to-day living, as it tends to occur over a longer period of time. In generalised anxiety, there are no specific triggers that set off a bout of anxiety; generally everything has the potential to make sufferers feel anxious.

These are the medical definitions, but when we discuss anxiety with our clients, we tend to use a slightly different explanation, which we think is easier to put into the context of what people are actually experiencing. We see anxiety as:

An emotional response to our own thoughts or thought processing.

Deep, right?

Let's explain. We all automatically assume that those anxious feelings come about because of something that has happened. But this is not strictly true. We believe there are a huge amount of thought processes that go on before we get to this emotional response. If we change our thought processes, we can effectively change the emotional response.

Now that we've established what anxiety is, let's look at how to control it and use it to our benefit.

ANXIETY CAN BE A POSITIVE THING

It's a fact that we all get anxious – it's part of everyday life. It's highly unlikely you've never felt nervous about a date or an interview. Often, this becomes a positive force, heightening our senses, focussing the mind and helping us perform at a higher level.

WHEN DOES IT BECOME A NEGATIVE?

When tears start falling, anger sets in and the anxious feelings take control. A lot of specialists say 'in order to deal with an anxiety attack just breathe, count to ten and stay calm'. If you are an anxiety sufferer, then you know that this is easier said than done – and that it also comes a little bit late when you're feeling out of control.

HOW TO GET ANXIETY WORKING ON OUR SIDE

What we want to do is make ourselves bulletproof to the triggers that set off an attack.

Say you want to join the gym, and you decide that tomorrow is going to be the day! Then six months pass by, you never join and now feel like you never will, and just the mere thought of the gym makes you feel 'urggh'. What happened? When you decided to take action (in this case, when you made the decision to join the gym) your brain went, 'OH MY GOD, WHAT IF? CHANGE!' When you think about the fact that you're joining the gym tomorrow, your heart rate rises a little, maybe your hands get clammy and you feel nervous. Naturally, your brain is going to say, 'wait a minute...hold up, this doesn't feel right. I don't like this feeling' and goes into full protection mode. It will also start playing out all the potential bad and good things that could happen, making you question whether or not going is a good idea. Our brains are naturally wired to think of more negatives than positives when it comes to the unknown, unless we train it otherwise. This is because our primal brain doesn't naturally deal with new things that have an uncertain outcome very well. We have evolved as a species in so many ways, but the ol' thinking box upstairs just hasn't kept up.

Nine times out of ten, we don't have the inner strength and belief to question ourselves and, very quickly, the negative thoughts start to outweigh the positives. Before we know it, we've talked ourselves out of whatever it was and carry on just as we always have done. Stepping outside our comfort zone is extremely hard, but in order to overcome battles in daily life and achieve long-term happiness we must take that step (see pages 38–39).

A simple way to help you think more rationally and positively is to start by writing a list of the potential positives and negatives about the situation you are feeling anxious about. Using the idea of going to the gym as an example, your list might start off looking a bit like this:

POSITIVES:
Get healthier
Feel better
Have more confidence

NEGATIVES:
I might hate it
It will be hard
People might laugh at me

Keep going, thinking of as many as you can. What you will start to notice is that when you spend some proper time thinking about it, if it's something you really want to do, the positives will outweigh the negatives and most of your negatives will be assumption-based rather than factual statements. Whereas your positive list will be full of strong facts and things that you want to achieve, which will instantly make you feel a little better.

If that process has worked for you and reassured you, then great; if not, then what next? Sometimes feeling anxious is so deeply set into our day-to-day life that we take a bit more convincing. This can be for many reasons – maybe a past trauma that felt similar to how you are feeling now, or maybe you just have a very vivid imagination. Time to bring out the big guns! Visualise the situation so that it becomes familiar and strips power from the negatives.

Take a seat on your favourite sofa or your bed, grab your favourite (preferably non-alcoholic!) drink and just stop. Turn off the TV, leave

'ANXIETY IS ONE CARD IN A HUGE DECK,
BUT REMEMBER WHO'S HOLDING THEM.'

the phone alone and close your eyes. Just concentrate on breathing slowly and steadily. After a couple of minutes, or whenever you feel completely relaxed, start to walk through the situation you're feeling anxious about in your mind. Imagine walking through the gym door, talking to the receptionist, signing up etc. There will be certain parts of the process that feel harder than others and you will start to identify little triggers that you have, which will be great for future reference – make sure to note them down. Try doing this a few times imagining different scenarios.

Walking through the situation in your head will make the real thing seem more familiar and less strange when you actually do it. This will leave you in a position whereby joining the gym is almost like being on autopilot – it's easy! You can concentrate on the important things, like *whoa, that machine looks strange, look at the size of that dude*, and so on.

This is a simple visualisation technique to help you with everyday anxious feelings or potential future situations that could stop you in your tracks. It will start to show you just how OVER THE TOP your mind can be at times.

Dealing with anxiety long term is very much like training, apart from the fact that it's internal. It's 'innercising' rather than exercising. But it's so important that you learn to deal with anxiety before it even becomes an issue.

Another practical method that helps a lot of people is planning in time every day to allow yourself to worry or stress as much they want. Sounds crazy, right? But stay with us. During the day, whenever you feel anxious, stressed or generally just 'arggh!' make a note of it, writing down what it was and why, then as you put it to one side tell it 'I'll deal with you later'. Then, decide on a fifteen-minute slot in your day and designate it your Worry Time. Make it the same time every day and a few hours before bed. So if you go to bed at 10 p.m., make it 6–6.15 p.m. Take a comfy seat and let it all out. Read through your notes, let the feelings rise again if they need to, and assess them all. Give them all airtime and just breathe through it. The first thing you will probably notice when you look back at that stressful event is that it was nowhere near as bad as it felt in that moment earlier in the day when you made the note. This process also teaches you to take control back from your anxiety by giving it a time to be there, but only when you say so. Over time you will notice that by adding that quick 'I'll deal with you later' will instantly start to relax the mind. Let your anxiety know that you've listened and are aware of its presence but now is not the time. Soon you will train your mind to know when is the time and place to worry, and when is not.

In summary, feeling anxious is actually quite an important thing to feel during tasks and new activities. It shows that we care about the outcome and – more importantly – it shows that we care about ourselves. Feeling anxious can be a problem if it holds us back from doing what we want, or we let it take over, so don't let that happen! Prepare yourself, strip away any thought that isn't factual, enter your inner cinema every now and then for a good ol' laugh, and give it all airtime. Embrace your fears and worries but always remember to filter out anything that isn't useful and beneficial to you. And finally, remember it is an ongoing process. Train your mind as hard as you train your body; a beautiful physique is only as beautiful as the mind behind it. We want you all to LOVE what you have.

LEARN TO BALANCE ⚖️

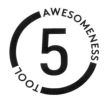

Let's take more of a look at this beautiful word we like to use so much: balance. What is the importance of balance and how do we strike it just right? Think of balance simply as a set of old-fashioned scales. On one side we want you to put your training, nutrition, work and anything else that requires you to literally take energy away from your body or brain. This is the external side of the scale – those activities that are external pulls on your time. The other side is where all the magic happens: time with your family, seeing your friends, resting, sleep, hobbies – basically all the stuff you do (or want to do) in your free time. We call these the internal factors – the activities that nourish you inside.

What so many of us don't do enough of is take time for ourselves. Quite simply, if you want to train hard and work hard all day, then that's great – but do not take it home with you. We know this is easier said than done, but try taking just a few baby steps to start with.

If we constantly over-stimulate our bodies but do not allow time to recover properly and regulate internally, our scales will start to tip and our stress levels will start to creep up higher. Our sleep will be affected, we can become agitated, experience brain fog, feel unable to concentrate and end up chronically fatigued or find ourselves constantly picking up colds and infections. This is your body telling you to stop, take time to recover and regulate. Sound like you?

It's a simple fix really.

Take a look back at your answers to the questionnaires earlier on in the chapter. What did you write down for 'What do you do for fun?' Make the decision today to do more of the things that you enjoy and find more time to relax. If you do that, every single other part of your life will improve and you'll feel more balanced. Even if you start off with something as simple as taking a relaxing bath, reading your favourite book for half an hour or aiming to get to bed thirty minutes earlier than you currently do to help your sleep improve.

When we talk about balance, let's quickly talk about having a few drinks and a good old knees-up with friends. So many people say to us, 'You're personal trainers, you can't drink alcohol!' We just utter one word in response. Know what it is? Yep, balance! We train hard and look after our bodies, so if we choose to go out and socialise with friends over a few drinks, then that's what we're going to do. It's so easy to obsess over everything related to health and fitness, but too much of anything just isn't good for you, and that goes for training too. Becoming obsessive about it is just as unhealthy as not caring in the slightest. Start striking that perfect balance of energy out and energy in and you will fly... well, not literally, but you know what we mean.

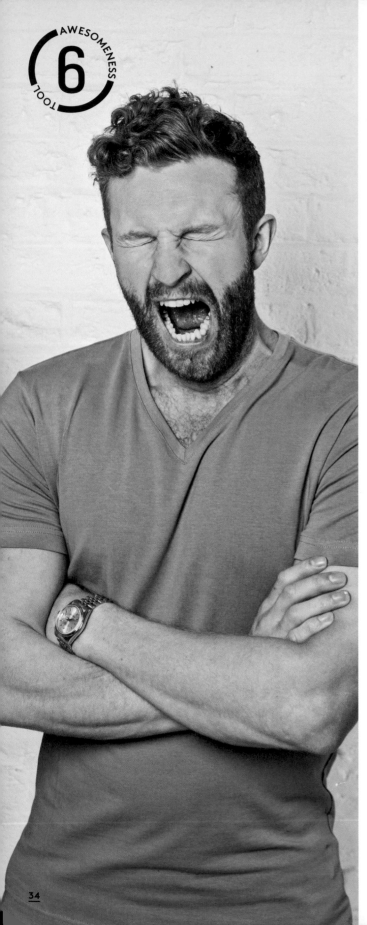

GET YOUR SLEEP SORTED

When it comes to increasing overall happiness and addressing issues of anxiety, overeating or lack of energy, very often the problems can be fixed if you GET YOUR SLEEP SORTED! A good eight hours a night will help the body do its thang internally and get you recovered and ready to go.

Sleep is crucial for health and performance and also helps you to learn new skills. You put your body under a lot of stress in the gym, but you repair and grow stronger outside the gym and it's important to get enough sleep to do this properly. When you are sleeping your body is repairing both physically and mentally. We also have peak concentrations of certain hormones through the night. While you sleep your brain is also preparing new pathways, helping you to learn and remember all the cool stuff you read in this book!

Eight hours of sleep is a good aim for most of us, although in the summer you may find you need a bit less and in the winter a bit more. Find out what you need and try and stick to it every night – even at the weekend.

BUT I CAN'T SLEEP!

Many of us struggle to either get to sleep or to stay asleep throughout the night. This is normally due to being stressed and with high levels of cortisol in your body. Cortisol is one of your primary stress hormones and should be higher in the morning to help you wake up as sunlight shines through your eyelids and stimulates its release. So if it's high at night you will most likely struggle to sleep. There are many reasons for this, from stimulation from light-emitting electrical devices (yes, that means your phone) to stress and even low blood sugar levels and hunger.

Feel like you can't sleep? Okay, so how do you prepare for your night's sleep? Like everything, it's all in the preparation. Here are some great ways to help you get off to the land of nod.

① **Turn off all electrical devices two hours before bedtime.** Those emails, the next episode on Netflix and Soda Crush can wait. You can do little about your work from your bed, and it will keep your brain busy when you should be shutting down. The light that shines from electrical devices also plays havoc with your stress hormones, making it harder to go to sleep and stay asleep all night.

② **Avoid caffeine** after 5 p.m., as it will still stimulate you long after you have had that initial whoosh and has the potential to delay your body clock.

③ **Get yourself into a bedtime routine** and start getting ready for bed around the same time each day. Give yourself plenty of time to do so – an hour is a good amount of time to aim for. Soon your body will start to recognise what's coming and will start to relax.

④ **Read a book or meditate before bed.** This allows your brain to unwind and stop thinking about work (see page 25 for our meditation techniques).

⑤ If you're feeling anxious about the day ahead and are struggling to switch off your work brain, get a notepad and write a list of simple bullet points of the important things that you have to do tomorrow. This will get them off your mind – you can deal with them in the morning.

⑥ **Most importantly, write a list of five things you are grateful for.** This will help you to fall asleep feeling content while thinking about them. Things like 'I am grateful for my supportive family', 'I'm grateful that I'm healthy', or even (and our favourite) 'I am grateful for the Mexican food I had for dinner.'

These are all very simple things to help the body start to shut down and concentrate on one thing – sleeping. Sleep is crucial in achieving happiness and the body you want, so treat it as part of your training and nutrition routine. Prepare for it properly and take the time to unwind before sleep. You will be amazed at how good you feel after a restful, quality night's sleep.

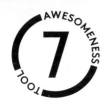

STOP REACTING TO EXTERNAL FORCES

'FOR EVERY MINUTE YOU ARE ANGRY, YOU LOSE SIXTY SECONDS OF HAPPINESS.' RALPH WALDO EMERSON

This is one of the earliest things we learnt, thanks to our mindset coach, Stephen Aish. It reminds us that we shouldn't react to external forces that are not meant for us. Stephen explained this to us with this good example:

Imagine you're on your computer, phone or tablet and suddenly your Wi-Fi kicks out. In a rage you throw out a few expletives. But it was not a personal attack on you. Do you think the big man up in the clouds went 'Hmm, you know what I want to do today? I want to mess around with John and Leon's Wi-Fi. That will really upset them.' Highly unlikely, right? These things will happen – and often do – but to lose your mind over them is madness.

Another one is another driver cutting you up, meaning you have to hit the brakes. Instead of keeping your cool (and your happiness) you go thermo-nuclear and punch the horn, wave your fist and offer them out on the hard shoulder of the motorway while your kids are in the back seat. Now this is an exaggeration for most of us, but it happens, and for all you know the car in front cut in because he was on the way to an emergency or because his wife was in labour.

We are not the centre of the earth; sometimes things won't go our way and our days will be disrupted. The real trick is to retain your cool and happiness when this happens. Next time something like this happens, play the game we play, which is to see how little you can let it affect you – just as if it bounces right off you. If you get cut up in the car, just try to smile and say 'that was a nice one' and make into a kind of joke. This stops you getting angry and helps maintain your cool and therefore your happiness.

DOUBT KILLS MORE DREAMS THAN FAILURE EVER WILL

SUZY KASSEM

TAKE A STEP OUTSIDE YOUR COMFORT ZONE – IT'S FUN OUT THERE!

> 'YOUR TRUE POTENTIAL BEGINS AT THE END OF YOUR COMFORT ZONE.' NEALE DONALD

This is an awesome statement. But come on, let's all be honest right now, how many times have you seen this come up on social media or heard someone say it to you and you just thought to yourself: here we go again... somebody else making me feel crap and like I'm underachieving.

We've both been there but now we can look back and understand a lot more about why it made us feel that way. When we saw this quote for the first time our first thought (after thinking the above) was, 'Well, that's great but how do I know what my comfort zone is and where it ends, where my true potential starts and how I get there?' Feeling disheartened and overwhelmed, we forgot about the quote and what it said and carried on in our little bubble as before.

So, let's have a deeper look at what your comfort zone is and why you should sometimes take a leap of faith and step outside of it.

Your comfort zone is that sweet spot in life, the friendships you may have purely because it's easier that way, the job that you know exactly how much you need to do to keep the boss off your back and to draw a wage each month, or maybe even being with someone because you don't know what you would do on your own.

Are you that person that at about 5 p.m. on a Sunday says, 'Urgh, the weekend is almost over and then it's back to work.' Do you pick on poor old Monday because he's associated with going to the office? If so, don't you want to be that person who is excited to go to work because you love it? Hand on heart, we honestly love our jobs. Yes, we work very long hours and, yes, sometimes we feel like we could do with a day off here and there, but those days are few and far between. We'd personally rather earn a lot less money and be happy than be rich and miserable.

We know this sounds pretty harsh but in order to really fly in life (whatever flying is to you), you really need to look at what's going on around you and how it makes you feel.

- If you want to be the boss of your boss or even of their boss, what's stopping you?
- If you want to travel the world and live out of a backpack, what's stopping you?
- If you want to lie around in your pyjamas all day and watch TV, what's stopping you?

Okay, maybe not that last one, but really, what is actually stopping you? That warm, squidgy cocoon-like place in your life called Comfort, as well as that big bad wolf called Fear. Fear is an extremely powerful feeling to have in your armoury; most of us see it as a negative emotion and run away from it so we don't enrage the beast within. But facing your fears can be a good thing! Here's another statement that really helped us understand what fear really is:

> As babies we are born with only two fears: the fear of falling and the fear of loud noises. Everything else we pick up along the way.

This short sentence was one of the first things Leon heard after embarking on his mindset journey. It really sunk in and has stuck with him ever since. He calls it his 'light bulb moment'.

In order to truly succeed in whatever area you want to improve, fears have to be met head-on and channelled in a positive way. First and foremost, it's as simple as understanding that fear is also a positive emotion. This will really help you to strip away the negativity you naturally associate it with in order to protect yourself. Fear, like its cousin anxiety (see pages 30–32), only ever holds the power you give it. Strip the power, strip the fear.

Facing fears on a daily, monthly or even yearly basis will show you your true potential. Of course, it's not a simple case of 'bye bye comfort zone, hello true potential', but if you're facing your fears and gaining experience – and smiling along the way – then never underestimate just how far you've already come and imagine where you could end up!

Let's finish up with a question from motivational speaker, Les Brown:

> 'Where's the wealthiest place on earth?'

Most will say, 'Err, Dubai? USA? Singapore?'

Well, the answer is actually the graveyard, because there lies all the unwritten songs and poems, the genius ideas, the broken hearts, the potential happiness – all because people were too scared to let their AWESOMENESS out. Please don't let that be you. You are amazing and you have so much to offer others, whether you are the person that gives a smile to someone in need or you create a lifesaving vaccine. The human race has survived because we can work as a team. Happiness isn't found in piles of money; it's found in your children's laughter, shared gestures and the warmth you feel from doing something utterly selfless. We can attest to this after working with WaterAid in Zambia; the happiness you bring to a community by helping them is just magical, and it's more fulfilling than any number of 0s in your bank account. It gives your life purpose.

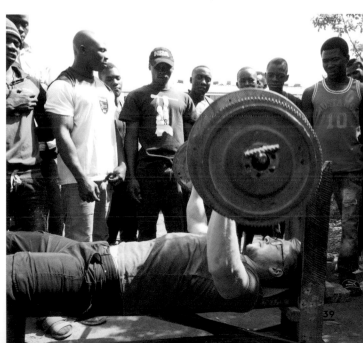

MAKE HAPPINESS YOUR MAIN GOAL

Life tends not to follow the happy-ever-after we expect from watching films when we were kids. Events will come out of the blue and knock you for six. The best-laid plans will fall apart and you'll have to constantly reassess your goals and your path through life. It's how you deal with those setbacks and general day-to-day stresses and bounce back from them that will have the most impact on your happiness.

Happiness should be your main goal in life. Tied into this are smaller goals – fitness, health, work, family, personal goals – but if you look at each of those areas and spend some time working on them, then happiness will follow.

Start small – maybe by using just one of the tools in this chapter – and very soon you'll feel inspired to use them all. And avoid reaching for quick fixes like junk food or booze to make you feel better. Work on the root causes of your happiness, make some simple lifestyle changes and start to feel AWESOME!

Happiness isn't tied to how much you earn, what you look like or where you live: it's a state of mind. And if all else fails, on those really bad days, boost your happiness with a good song or film that will remind you of what's really important in life.

Here are some of our favourites:

FILMS	SONGS
THE BUCKET LIST	FOLLOW THE SUN by XAVIER RUDD
HECTOR AND THE PURSUIT OF HAPPINESS	L.I.F.E.G.O.E.S.O.N. by NOAH AND THE WHALE
ABOUT TIME	MOVE HOW YOU WANT by BEN HOWARD
THE PEACEFUL WARRIOR	EVERYBODY'S FREE (TO WEAR
UP	SUNSCREEN) by BAZ LUHRMANN
STEP BROTHERS	3 LITTLE BIRDS & COULD YOU BE LOVED
	by BOB MARLEY AND THE WAILERS

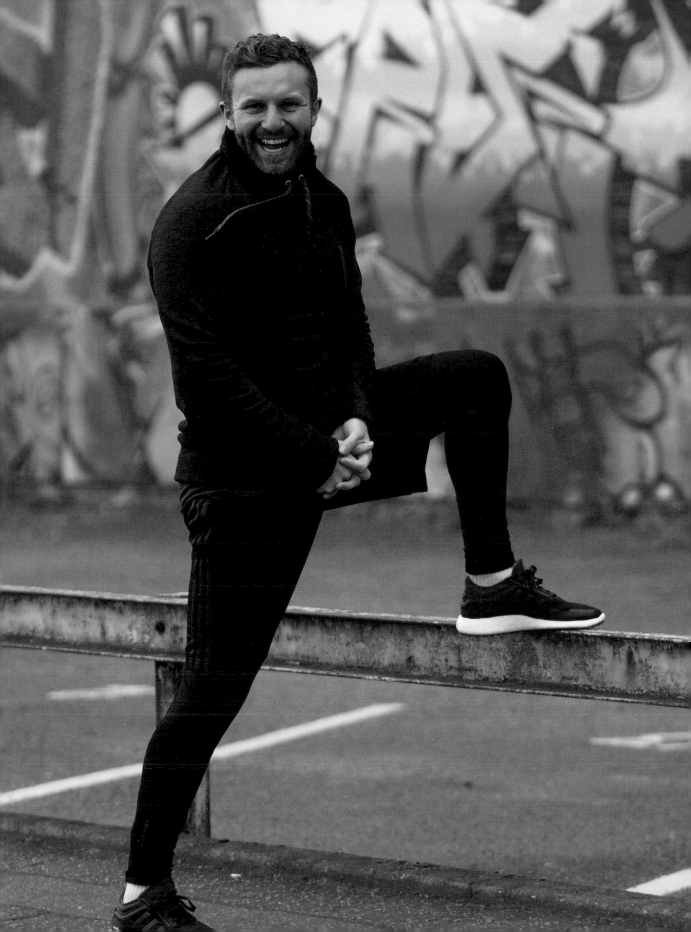

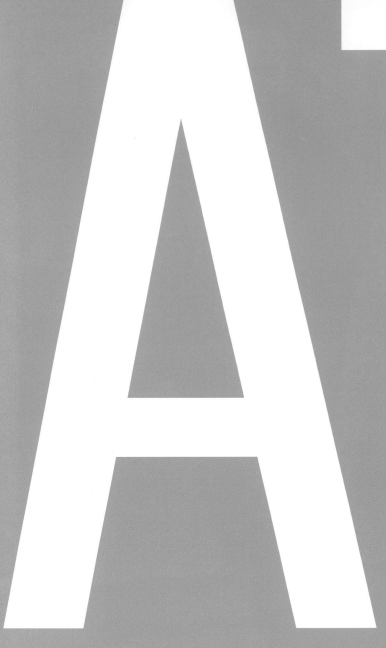

EAT

It's time to learn how to start shaping your ideal body and know what it's like to feel healthy and awesome. This chapter is going to teach you exactly what you need to eat and, most importantly, why. It's time to stop listening to the gym bros and your friend of a friend for poor advice. These methods and recipes are tried and tested; we use them on a daily basis.

We want to teach you the basics: how many calories should you be eating for your goals, and where should they come from? Once you've learned how to work these out, we have 60 awesome recipes with the calorie count and macronutrients already worked out for you, so you can eat delicious food that's great for you.

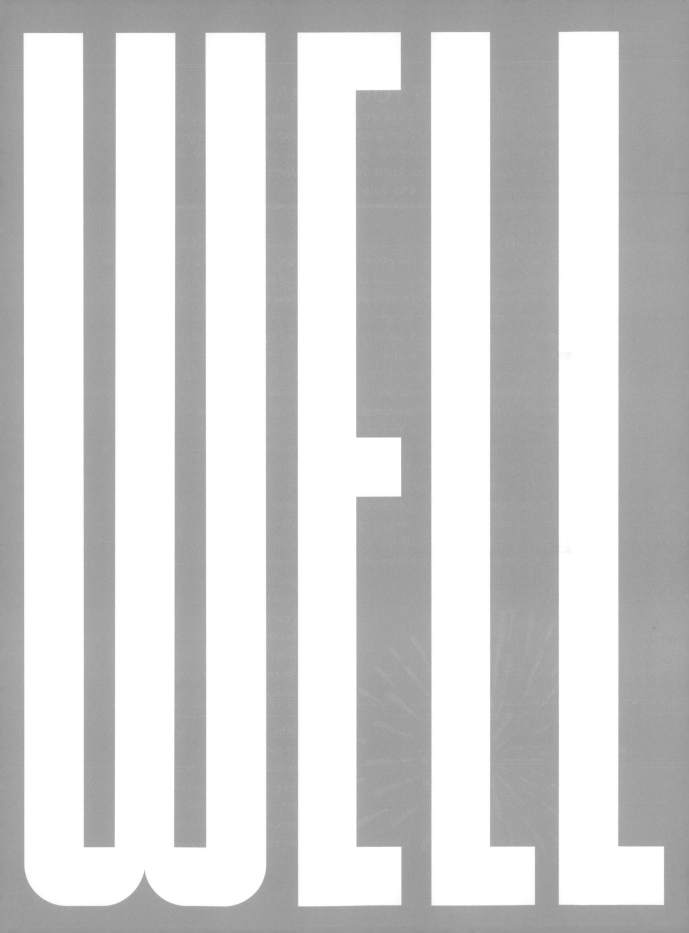

STEP ①: WHAT IS YOUR GOAL?

What you eat will largely dictate your appearance, your health and your performance. Body composition goals are governed by energy balance – eating the correct amount of calories for your goals in conjunction with your activity levels is the single most important factor in whether you will lose fat, gain muscle or even gain fat. It's the foundation.

FAT LOSS

This is a very common goal, and all too often it is mislabelled as 'weight loss'. Weight loss is a vague term and could imply losing a mixture of fat, muscle, glycogen and water. Muscle is metabolically active, which means it actually *uses* calories. Water is crucial for hydration. Ideally, the only thing you want to lose is fat. Fat can often be perceived as unattractive, but more important than that, it's associated with many health risks. The ideal way to diet is slowly, as it's more sustainable; the slower you diet the more you will be able to hold on to that all-important and hard-earned muscle. Remember, a good diet is a diet you can stick to. To lose fat, you need to consume less energy than you expend to create a caloric deficit. A great fat loss target is to lose 1-3 lb per week.

MUSCLE GAIN

We want – no – we *need* you to understand that building muscle is healthy and important. We know many women often worry about getting bulky – but that's just not likely as you produce so little testosterone compared to us guys and even we find it very hard to build muscle. It would take a long time and a lot of hard work before you ever felt 'too big' – we've never had a client who has said she feels this way. In fact, clients often feel bulky to start with due to having a higher percentage of body fat, and much less muscle. Our point is: don't be scared of working your butt off in the gym or at home by incorporating some heavy lifts. We one-hundred per cent recommend it, especially if you want to improve your posture, lose that extra fat and build that body shape that you aspire to. Plus, the more muscle you have, the more food you can eat when dieting – who doesn't want that, right? Building muscle requires that we exercise correctly and are in an energy surplus: this quite simply means we need to consume more energy than we are expending.

A healthy muscle gain is ¼-½lb per week. If you aim for more, you will undoubtedly gain more fat too and potentially no more muscle. It takes patience not to ramp up the calories too fast, but building muscle is a slow process that requires a lot of time in the gym – you need to learn to love it!

STEP ②: HOW MUCH SHOULD YOU EAT?

Everyone's body is different. The easiest way to work out how many calories you need to eat a day to achieve your goals is to first find out your BMR (basal metabolic rate) using a formula such as the Harris-Benedict formula via an online calculator. Your BMR is the amount of calories your body needs just to function at rest. It's the energy needed to keep your organs working and equates to roughly sixty per cent of your total calories, or your TDEE (total daily energy expenditure). This is the amount of calories your body burns in a day, based on your BMR plus activity levels. Use the formula below to work out your TDEE to give you an idea of how many calories you need daily to maintain your weight.

WRITE YOUR BMR HERE: **KCAL/DAY**

Now you know your BMR, you need to factor in your daily activity. You can work this out as follows (or use an online calculator):

BMR x 1.2   for low-intensity activities and leisure activities (primarily sedentary)

....

BMR x 1.375   for light exercise, such as leisurely walking for 30–50 minutes, 3–4 days per week

....

BMR x 1.55   for moderate exercise 3–5 days per week

....

BMR x 1.725   for active individuals exercising 6–7 days per week

....

BMR x 1.9   for extremely active individuals engaged in heavy/intense exercise, such as heavy manual labour, heavy lifting, endurance athletes and competitive team sports athletes 6–7 days per week

This formula will give you an idea of your TDEE but remember, we are all very different with different lifestyles, so for some it may actually work out too low and for others too high.

To lose fat you need to create a safe calorie deficit. In theory, a weekly calorie deficit of 3,500 equates to 1lb of fat loss per week. This means cutting 500 calories per day off your TDEE. This deficit can be created by more exercise, fewer calories, or a combination of both! Often the bulk of this deficit would come from carbs, as protein and fat are essential macronutrients. If you have worked out your TDEE and your goal is fat loss, you can now remove calories to create your deficit – this is your new TDEE. The higher your body fat percentage and the closer you are to being obese, the more calories you may need to remove from your TDEE. This is due to the BMR calculation using your weight in the formula BUT fat does not burn calories like muscle. For a more accurate TDEE use a calculator that uses your lean body mass such as The Katch-McArdle Formula (NOTE: you will need to know your body fat percentage for this).

To gain weight you need to increase your calories and train effectively in the gym. Remember the phrase progressive overload: this simply means you must keep progressing for your body to adapt, whether that's more reps, more weight or more volume to build muscle.

STEP ③ : KNOW YOUR MACROS!

There are three main macronutrients that we need to consume, and they all have different energy values, effects and requirements in our bodies

Note: alcohol does not count as a macronutrient – it provides no nourishment, only headaches.

CARBOHYDRATE

Carbohydrates can be broken down into two types: simple carbs and complex carbs. Quite simply, simple carbs are faster absorbed than complex carbs. We know this because of a scale called the GI scale or Glycaemic Index, which was created for people with diabetes to understand how certain foods would affect their blood sugar levels. The closer a carbohydrate's rating is to 100, the faster it is absorbed and enters the bloodstream. We want to utilise both high GI and low GI carbs, but we can be a bit more intelligent about it.

As a general rule we use our higher GI carbs after or during training to allow for better performance, recovery and to take advantage of certain processes that happen in the body after exercise. At this time your body is primed and ready to be refuelled and replace used glycogen. Glycogen is the stored form of glucose, a major fuel source for the body and what most carbohydrates get broken down into before they enter our bloodstream.

Ideally these higher GI carbs should still come from good sources, where possible. We know lots of people drink things like chocolate milk after training, and if there is a time to drink it, it's then! Still, there are healthier options such as bananas.

Simple carbohydrates are found naturally in foods like milk and fruits; they are also found in processed foods such as sweets, fizzy drinks, syrups, table sugar and white bread.

Complex carbs are things like sweet potatoes, brown rice, basmati rice and most vegetables, especially leafy greens and most nuts.

Many people, including us, have used low-carb diets before. For us that meant less than 100–150g a day. Many people think this may help you lose body fat, as it will decrease spikes in blood sugar (glucose) and thus insulin. Insulin is the hormone that your pancreas releases when your blood sugar is raised. This is to help you store the blood sugar (glucose) from the carbs you eat into your cells. But it also puts the brakes on fat-burning for a short time, so if you're about to do cardio with fat loss in mind, then sugary isotonic drinks will raise your blood sugar and halt fat-burning. The jury is still out on the effectiveness of low-carb diets due to fewer insulin spikes; this is because protein alone will still raise insulin levels.

We feel that fat loss achieved by low-carb dieting is often largely due to consuming less calories. It also has the drawback of cutting out a major food group, which is hard to do and leaves little variety in your diet. Also, remember that glucose is the major fuel source for your body and especially your brain, so sometimes you can get grouchy and find it hard to focus.

As a whole, this diet lacks balance as a long-term solution in our opinion; however, it may be used intelligently to reduce body fat, or in the pre-diabetic population to restore insulin sensitivity.

There is always the option of carb cycling, which we often use. On days when we are training hard or we need more energy for performance, our carbs will be higher; on days of no training and less activity, we will have fewer carbs. This gives us the best of both worlds and allows us to switch between using fat or carbs as a primary fuel source more efficiently. This is known as metabolic flexibility.

PROTEIN

Protein is responsible for rebuilding and repairing the tissues of our body, such as muscle, nails and hair. It also plays important roles with hormones, enzymes and the immune system. Protein is made up of amino acids, the building blocks of protein, and you will get different amino acids from an array of foods. Meat is considered the main source of complete protein, as it contains all the essential amino acids. Essential amino acids cannot be synthesised by the body and therefore must be acquired through a varied diet, while non-essential amino acids can be synthesised by the body. So meat is a great choice for a complete protein, but you can also mix up lots of foods that are not 'complete' to still get all the required essential amino acids.

If you are vegan or vegetarian, don't panic! You still have plenty of choices for really good-quality protein sources, such as quinoa, buckwheat, hempseed, chickpeas, beans, nuts and many more.

Protein is essential for everyone, especially those who partake in regular resistance training – and that means you now! Protein recommendations are set as low as 0.8g per kg of body weight – this is very low, even for sedentary individuals, so if you are looking to build muscle we suggest between 1.4–2.5g per kg for healthy individuals.

Women are usually better suited to lower ranges of around 1.4g per kg, as typically they have less muscle.

FAT

Fat contains the most calories per gram, and has had a bad press in recent years, which has led to many people avoiding it. Fat, like everything else, needs to be eaten in moderation. However, fat is NOT bad for you; we only need to worry about over-consumption of fat and certain types of artificial fat like trans fats (found in certain brands of margarine and hydrogenated vegetable oil), which the body does not recognise, and can raise the risk of coronary heart disease and inflammation in the body. You will be amazed at how many companies use trans fats as they are cheap and have a long shelf life, so be sure to keep an eye on what you buy (hey, that rhymed, we'll have to use that more often).

Saturated fat comes mostly from animal products like fattier meats, butter, cheese and cream. Notice that these products are solid at room temperature. Saturated fat creates cholesterol and primary sex hormones like testosterone, which again plays a big part in building muscle tissue and reducing body fat. Cholesterol is another misunderstood substance that has been given a bad rap in the past, but provided you are healthy and eat a decent diet, your liver will simply produce less cholesterol when you eat more of it. Your body is incredibly good at maintaining balance – this is known as homeostasis. We could spend a few pages just talking about cholesterol and its importance but we will save that for another day! If you want to know more, a great book to read is *The Great Cholesterol Con* by Dr Malcolm Kendrick.

Monounsaturated fats are known as 'good' fats and they are liquid at room temperature. They're found in nuts like cashews and peanuts, in avocados and many oils like olive oil. You definitely want adequate amounts of these in your diet.

Polyunsaturated Fats include the most talked about omega-3, omega-6 and omega-9, although there are plenty more. Omega-3 is found in oily fish like wild salmon and mackerel. It is probably the most beneficial to those of us with a western diet as it has anti-inflammatory properties and our diets are typically high in omega-6, which is pro-inflammatory. Omega-6 is also important but ideally, instead of trying to balance out the amount of omega-6 we eat with tons of omega-3, which is expensive, it may be more effective to educate ourselves on what our diet contains.

We recommend eating oily fish or even flax and chia seeds to get your dose of omega-3. A supplement may be used to up your intake; just make sure it's good-quality one as you get what you pay for and poor-quality versions may contain heavy metals like mercury.

FIBRE

Strictly speaking, this isn't a macronutrient, but we think it's very important. It is great for keeping you regular and helping reduce the risk of bowel disease. It's also really good for keeping you feeling full, which is handy if you're trying to lose fat. It's mainly found in complex carbs like grains and veg such as broccoli.

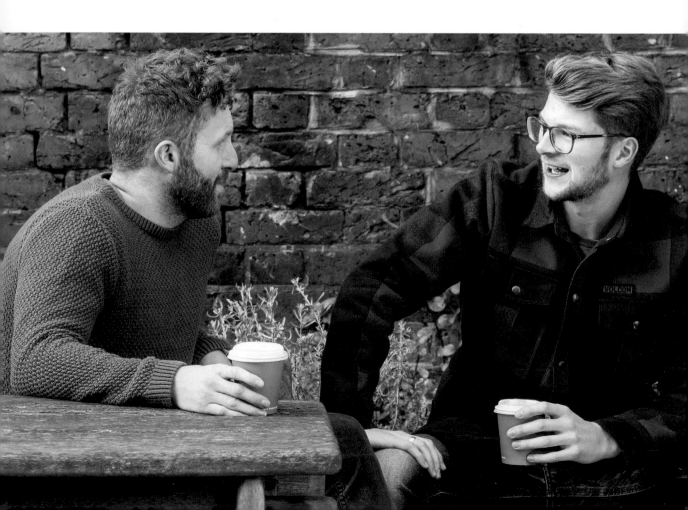

STEP ④: WHAT SHOULD YOU EAT?

Here are some guidelines for how much you should consume of each macronutrient based on your body weight. As always, this won't suit everybody, but it's a great starting point for you to monitor what works for you. If you are more active you will most likely require higher amounts of carbs than someone who is less active, so if you have a desk job and are rarely active apart from the gym, it may be wise to save the bulk of your daily carbs for times around your workout.

Once you've worked out your macros, you'll be able to calculate which of our recipes you should go for. The best way to work out how much of each macronutrient you're eating is to track your meals using an app such as MyFitnessPal, or to use our recipes – which have all the macros calculated for you!

Use these guidelines based on your own body weight for active individuals to work out how much of each macro you should be eating:

PROTEIN (4 kcal per gram)
1.4–2.5g protein per kg of body weight =
_____ g x 4 kcal = _____ kcal

CARBS (4 kcal per gram)
The rest of your day's calories should come from carbs

FAT (9 kcal per gram)
0.8–1.2g fat per kg of body weight =
_____ g x 9 kcal = _____ kcal

FIBRE!
Try to make sure you get about 10–14g fibre per 1,000 calories consumed

---

To make it easier, here's a step-by-step example of how John calculates his daily macros. Don't worry, it's not as complicated as it looks!

John's weight is 80kg and his TDEE shows he needs 2,925 kcal/day

He needs approx. 2g per kg of body weight of PROTEIN: 2g x 80 = 160g protein/day
Protein has 4 kcal/g, so 160 x 4 = 640 kcal/day

He needs approx. 1g per kg of body weight of FAT: 1g x 80 = 80g fat/day
Fat has 9 kcal/g, so 80 x 9 = 720 kcal/day

The rest of his calories need to come from carbs – his daily calorie allowance is 2,925

2925 – 640 (protein) – 720 (fat) = 1,565

He has 1,565 kcal left to have as carbohydrates, which is 4 kcal/g
Therefore, John's goal for carbs is 1,565g ÷ 4 = 391g carbs

So John's daily macros overall are as follows: 80g fat, 160g protein and 391g carbs

TRACKING YOUR FOOD

It's important to find out how food makes you feel. We both know John can easily consume 391g carbs a day and feel great, due to his body type, high activity levels and intensity of exercise. You, however, may find that once you work out your macros you need to tinker with them, for example if you're not as active as John or you feel bloated due to higher amounts of carbs, then you can reduce your carbs and increase your fat and/or protein to help balance this out. We are all different so find what works for you. There is typically an inverse relationship between carbs and fats, if one goes up the other normally comes down, while still hitting your calorie goals.

This would be the ideal point to start writing a food diary or using an app like MyFitnessPal. By tracking your intake for one week you will find out the average amount of calories you currently consume daily.

Start keeping a food diary of everything you eat and drink for one week. It's a great tool to review what you have been eating and what patterns arise. People are often shocked when they see how many naughty snacks they actually have in a week, or how many calories those milky coffees add up to.

You can also write down your moods and how you feel after meals, as this may give you a clue to what works for you. For example, if you have milk and find you feel bloated, need the loo or just don't feel great, you may not work well with lactose; this is something you can explore and possibly avoid. The same applies to the usual culprits of gluten and nightshades such as mushrooms and peppers. We are all different and we should listen to how our bodies respond to our diets. So many of us are used to feeling substandard that when we actually eat well and start to feel awesome, we finally start to find that certain foods may not agree with us.

Once you have finished your food diary you can carry on tracking your calories each day if you choose to. However, once you have a grasp on what foods contain, you may choose to listen to your body and keep your calories in check visually, depending on your goals and how confident you feel.

There can be downsides to tracking your food in the long term. It can be tedious and even unhealthy, so if you choose to count calories and macronutrients for long periods of time, make sure it's from a positive place where you control your food, and not from a negative place where your food is controlling you. But you HAVE to have a starting point as a reference to find out if your calorie targets are correct: calculations and calculators are rarely one-hundred per cent accurate and without being strict for a week or two and checking your results you will be just grasping at thin air. Even if you gain half a kilo instead of losing it, at least you know where you are in relation to your goals; you can then adjust by reducing your calories or increasing your exercise.

REMEMBER: not all calories are created equal. Picture 1,000 calories of chocolate vs. 1,000 calories of vegetables: not only do you get very different quantities of food, but they also have very different nutritional values. We want you to get more nourishment from your food than ever before, to allow you to feel great and for your body to perform and adapt.

STEP ⑤: THE IDEAL SHOPPING LIST

There are a few ingredients and products that we recommend you keep in your cupboards.

BUTTER - Ditch the low-fat spreads and margarine and stick with real butter! It's much tastier and better for you.

OILS - Virgin coconut oil is one of our favourite oils as it has a high content of MCTs (medium chain triglycerides), which are more readily used as energy. It's also very heat stable so is a great choice for frying. Olive oil is the main oil we use, ideally extra-virgin, which is great on salad and has many health benefits.

SEASONING - Get creative with your seasoning as variety is the spice of life!

GRASS-FED MEAT & FREE-RANGE EGGS - Aim to buy meat that is grass-fed, organic and/or free-range – including eggs – not only is it kinder to animals, it's also nutritionally much better for you.

GREEN VEGETABLES - These should be a huge part of your diet. They are full of nutrients, vitamins and antioxidants as well as being low calorie and high in fibre. Try to get some green veg in all of your meals.

NUTS - Are a great healthy snack, full of healthy fats and protein depending on your choice of nut. Beware not to eat too many as they can be quite calorific.

FROZEN BERRIES - Are awesome to chuck into smoothies. Not only are they high in antioxidants but they also act like ice cubes, making your smoothie much more appetising.

BOTTLED WATER - If you struggle to drink enough water each day, buy a big bottle and mark lines and times down the side with a permanent marker. For example, divide it into Breakfast, Midday, Afternoon and Night. This will help you drink enough water by having visible goals to hit throughout the day.

FREEZER & MICROWAVE-SAFE BAGS - Freeze soups or chillies in microwave-safe bags, laying them flat in the freezer. This means they will re-heat much faster in the microwave.

TUPPERWARE - If you don't have a kitchen at work or the budget to visit healthy food shops on your break, then you will need some decent containers so that you can prepare food in advance to take to work.

OILY FISH - Like mackerel, salmon and trout is a great addition to your shopping list as it has plenty of healthy fats, especially omega 3 which has a plethora of health benefits.

PULSES, LEGUMES & GRAINS - Are superb when it comes to fibre content. They also contain plenty of protein making them a great option, especially if you're vegetarian or vegan.

STEP ⑥: RULES TO REMEMBER

DON'T PANIC if you fall off the wagon! Just accept what's happened and get back on track as soon as you can. At worst you may set yourself back a week or two but just keep going. Remember, this is an ongoing process.

SUPPLEMENTS ARE JUST THAT

– a supplement to a good, varied diet. Some supplements, like caffeine, creatine, whey protein and fish oils, are great to include in a healthy, active lifestyle, but you need real food and a solid diet as the foundation; this will give you better results than any legal supplement.

SINGLE INGREDIENT FOODS.

The majority of the food you eat should be from single ingredient foods – natural foods like meat, fish and vegetables that haven't been processed. This means you will have to cook and prepare meals from scratch, which is pretty fun when you get into it – just stick on some tunes and get in the groove! You need to know exactly what is going into your body, so you can avoid the excess calories, junk and preservatives found in most ready-made meals.

PROTECT YOUR METABOLISM.

Crash, low-calorie diets will sting you in the long run: this is a lifestyle, not a race.

CALORIES are very important in your fat loss or muscle gain goals – but they need to come from foods that will support your health.

BE KIND TO YOUR GUT. Avoid chronic stress or stressors, like junk food, trans fats and inflammatory foods, alcohol and overuse of antibiotics, to name a few. You can also aid your gut health by consuming a diet rich in colourful vegetables, while fermented foods such as sauerkraut and yoghurt can also aid your intestinal flora.

DON'T FEAR CARBS. The 'no carbs after 6 p.m.' theory is a load of old rubbish, in our opinion. Your last meal before bed can certainly have carbs in it, it doesn't matter. What's important is that you hit your target calories and/or macros each day. Protein is the one macro you should really try to stay on top of when dieting – too low an intake along with a calorie deficit and you stand to lose muscle, which we know is not good. This is because your body will start to break down protein for fuel.

THE 80/20 RULE. We're not about eating like rabbits! The bulk of your food should be good and nutritious, but twenty per cent can be slightly less 'healthy', providing your calories are right for you and you are active. By allowing a little freedom you are more likely to avoid day-long over-eating binges.

BE PREPARED. Preparing your food ahead will help to eliminate the most common time we fall off the wagon – when we are caught short after a busy day and can't wait for the time it takes to prepare and cook a meal. Being prepared will stop you staving off hunger with easy foods like chocolate and crisps.

A NOTE ON MACROS:

The nutritional content of food varies from brand to brand and calories are often rounded up or down, so you may find that the macros we have provided for the recipes fall within about ten per cent of the total calories.

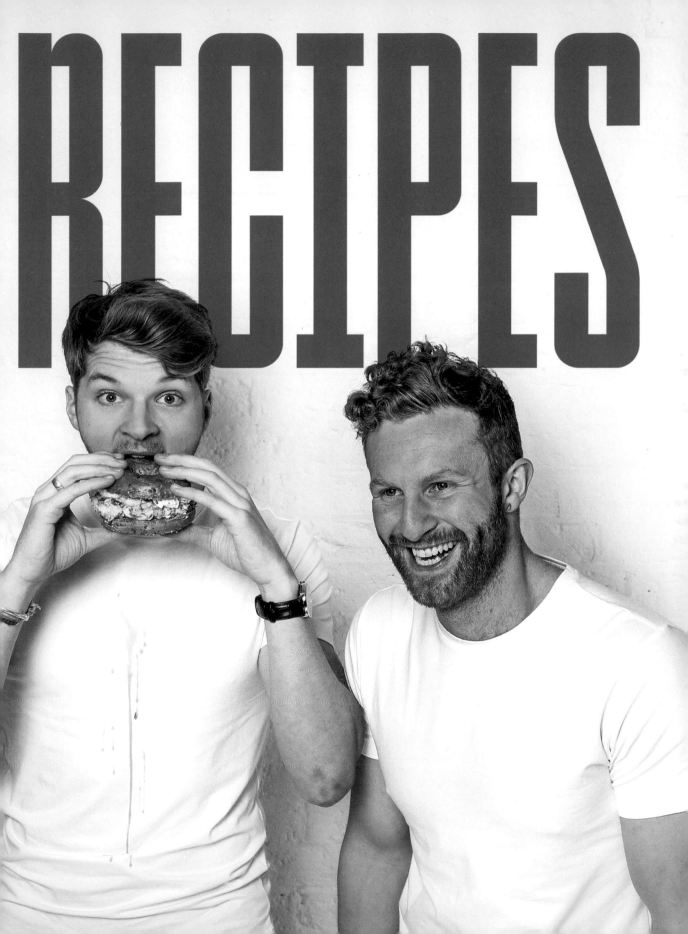

RECIPES

GET UP + GO SMOOTHIE

SMOOTHIES ARE BRILLIANT FOR THOSE WHO ARE SHORT ON TIME IN THE MORNING. THEY ALSO PROVIDE A GREAT OPPORTUNITY TO GET TONS OF NUTRIENTS AND VITAMINS INTO YOUR BODY IN ONE GO, NOT TO MENTION THE HEALTH BENEFITS OF THE FLAXSEED AND THE ANTIOXIDANT POWERS OF BERRIES. THIS IS A BALANCED SMOOTHIE WITH ADEQUATE AMOUNTS OF PROTEIN, FATS AND CARBS, MAKING IT IDEAL FOR ANY TIME OF THE DAY.

SERVES 1
100–200ml unsweetened almond milk
Handful of frozen blueberries (40g)
Handful of spinach leaves
6 frozen raspberries
25g rolled oats
1 scoop vanilla whey protein
    powder (30g)
1 tablespoon flaxseed
1 tablespoon chia seeds
1 tablespoon desiccated coconut
    (optional)

Combine all of the ingredients in a blender and whizz until smooth.

PER SERVING:
KCAL: 468   FAT: 16g
CARBS: 48g   PROTEIN: 33g

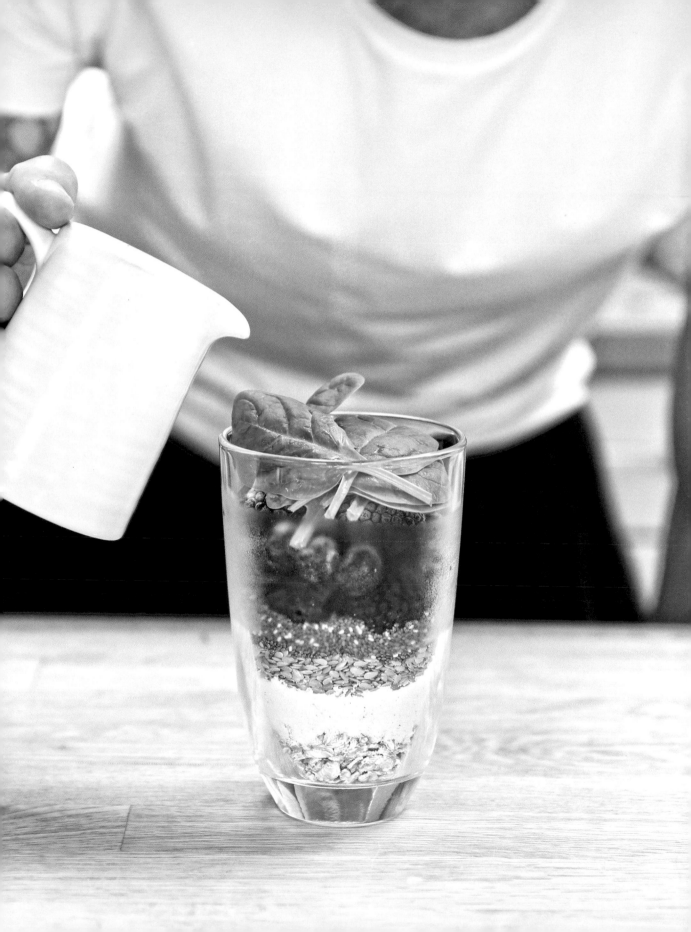

BREAKFAST SMOOTHIE

THIS SMOOTHIE IS LOW IN FAT AND HIGH IN CARBOHYDRATE AND PROTEIN, MAKING IT A GREAT CHOICE FOR AFTER YOUR MORNING WORKOUT – OR EVEN BEFORE IF BUILDING MAXIMUM MUSCLE IS YOUR GOAL. IF YOU'RE LOOKING FOR A SLIGHTLY LOWER CARB SMOOTHIE THEN LOSE THE DATES TO SAVE OVER 30G OF CARBS.

SERVES 1

200ml unsweetened almond milk

1 ripe banana, broken into chunks

6 fresh raspberries

2 Medjool dates, pitted

Pinch of ground cinnamon

1 scoop vanilla whey protein
  powder (30g)

Combine all of the ingredients in a blender and whizz until smooth.

PER SERVING:
KCAL: 429   FAT: 5g
CARBS: 72g   PROTEIN: 28g

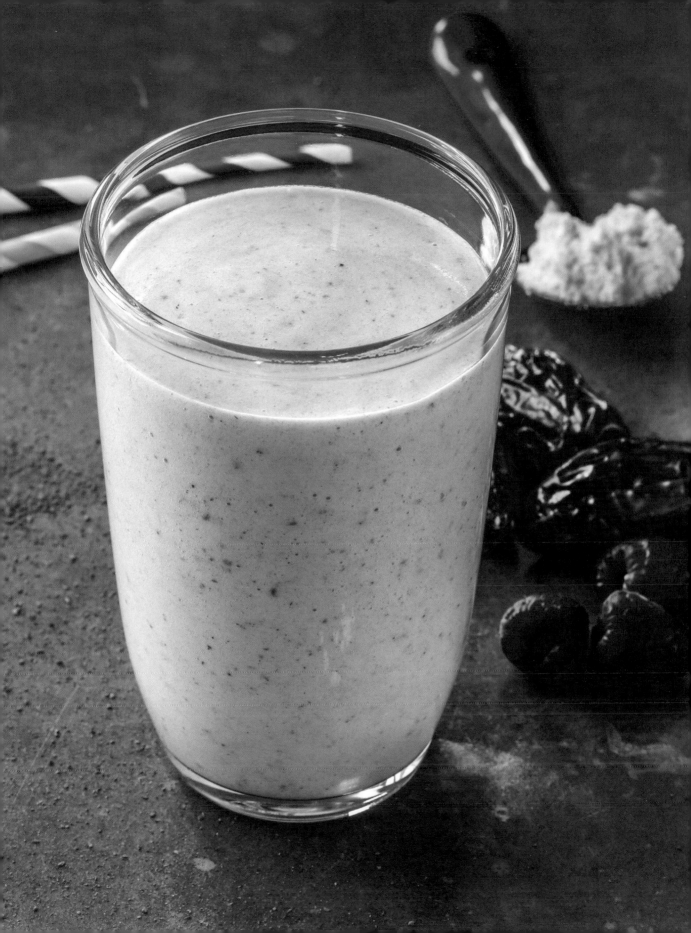

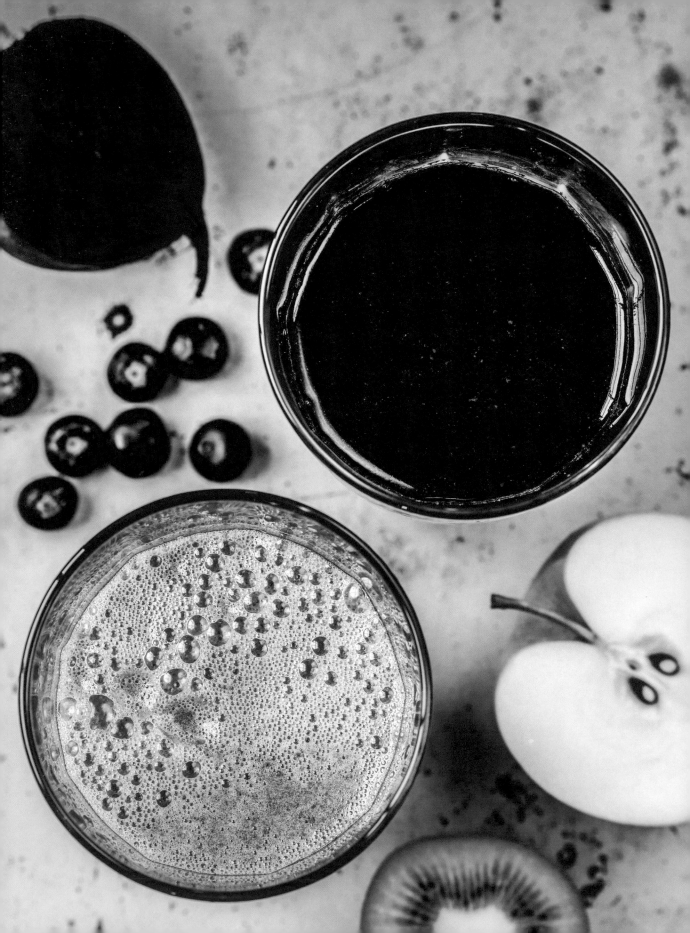

BEETROOT + BERRY JUICE

JUICES ARE THE SIMPLEST AND QUICKEST WAY TO GET A GOOD NUTRIENT BOOST AT THE START OF THE DAY – JUST DON'T GO TOO CRAZY WITH THE FRUIT OR YOU'LL SEND YOUR SUGAR LEVELS SOARING.

MAKES ABOUT 500ML – SERVES 1

1 large beetroot (120g), washed

1 apple, quartered and cored

1 medium carrot

150g blueberries

50g raspberries (fresh or frozen)

Juice of ½ lemon, or to taste

PER SERVING:
KCAL: <u>277</u>   FAT: <u>2g</u>
CARBS: <u>60g</u>   PROTEIN: <u>5g</u>

Cut the beetroot, apple and carrot into chunks small enough to fit into the neck of your juicer. Juice all of the ingredients except the lemon then stir to combine. Add lemon juice to taste.

If you don't have a juicer, tip all of the ingredients into a liquidiser and blend until smooth. Set a fine sieve over a large jug then pour the mixture in. Use the back of a ladle or a large spoon to push the mixture through, trapping the pulp and fibres in the sieve.

GREEN MACHINE SMOOTHIE

THINK OF THIS AS A BIT OF A HEALTHY ENERGY DRINK WITH A DECENT AMOUNT OF CARBS.

MAKES ABOUT 600ML – SERVES 2

2 Granny Smith apples, quartered
   and cored

½ cucumber

2 kiwi fruit, peeled

2 celery sticks

400g baby leaf spinach

Juice of ½ lemon, or to taste

PER 300ML SERVING:
KCAL: <u>186</u>   FAT: <u>2g</u>
CARBS: <u>35g</u>   PROTEIN: <u>7g</u>

Cut the apples, cucumber, kiwi fruit and celery into chunks small enough to fit into the neck of your juicer. Juice all of the ingredients except the lemon then stir to combine. Add lemon juice to taste.

If you don't have a juicer, tip all of the ingredients into a liquidiser and blend until smooth. Set a fine sieve over a large jug then pour the mixture in. Use the back of a ladle or a large spoon to push the mixture through, trapping the pulp and fibres in the sieve.

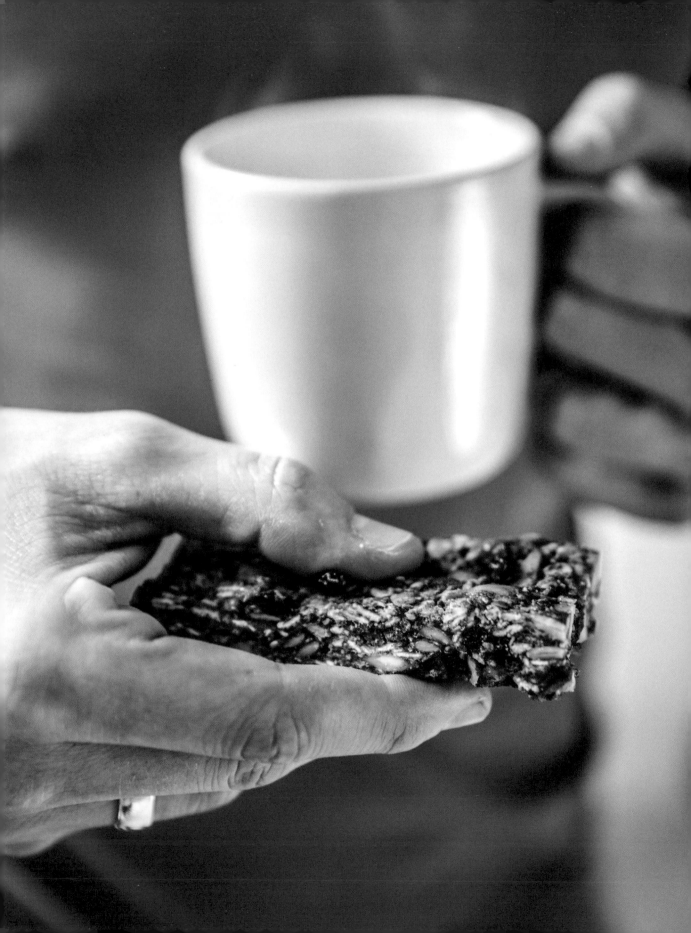

BREAKFAST BAR

THESE LITTLE BARS MAKE A GREAT BREAKFAST IF YOU'RE RUSHING OUT THE DOOR, BUT YOU CAN ALSO PACK THEM IN YOUR BAG AS A PERFECT POST-WORKOUT SNACK, PARTICULARLY WHEN EATEN WITH SOMETHING THAT WILL PROVIDE YOU WITH SOME GOOD PROTEIN, SUCH AS A WHEY SHAKE.

MAKES 12

12 Medjool dates, pitted

2 tablespoons almond butter

2 tablespoons coconut oil, melted

150g rolled oats

100g blanched almonds, roughly chopped

100g dried cranberries or dried cherries

50g puffed rice

50g pumpkin seeds

2 tablespoons chia seeds

2 tablespoons desiccated coconut

Put the dates into a small heatproof bowl, cover with boiling water and leave to stand for 10 minutes. Meanwhile preheat the oven to 150°C/gas mark 2 and line the base and sides of a 30x20cm cake tin with baking parchment.

Drain the dates, reserving the water, and put into a food processor with 100ml of the soaking water, the almond butter and coconut oil and blend until smooth. Combine the remaining ingredients in a large bowl, add the date mixture and stir to combine.

Press the mixture into the lined tin then bake for 40 minutes until golden brown around the edges. Remove from the oven and leave to cool in the tin.

Turn out onto a chopping board then use a serrated knife to cut into 12 equal rectangles. Wrap the bars individually in cling film then store in an airtight container. These freeze well so make a double batch and freeze half.

PER BAR:
KCAL: 280   FAT: 12g
CARBS: 39g   PROTEIN: 6g

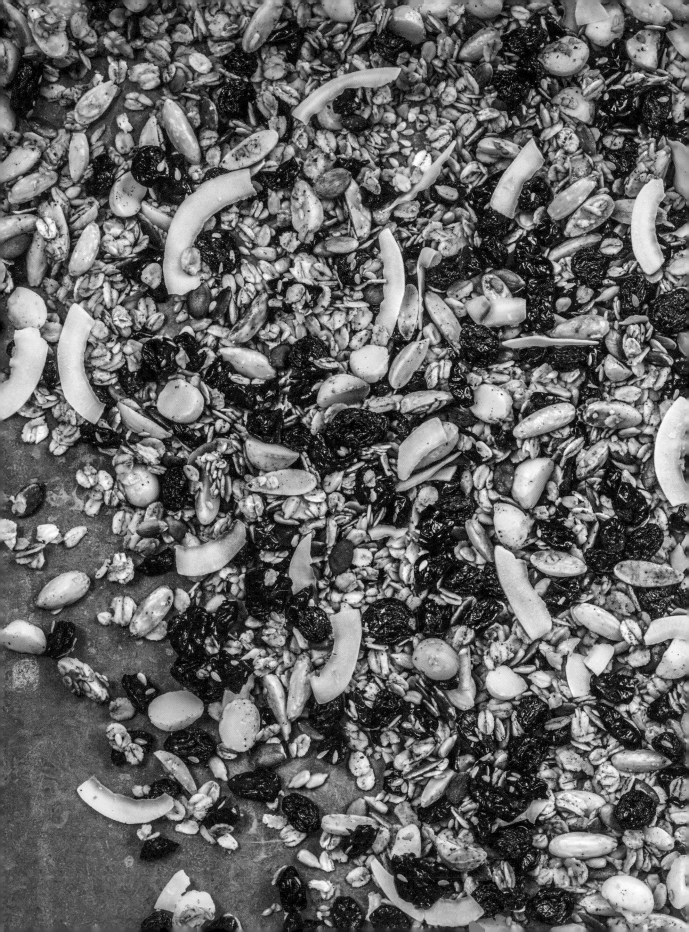

GRANOLA

GRANOLA IS A GREAT WAY TO GET IN EXTRA CALORIES AND LOTS OF GOOD FATS VIA NUTS AND SEEDS. WHEN SPLIT INTO 10 PORTIONS, THE PROTEIN CONTENT CAN BE A BIT LOW FOR THOSE WITH HIGHER DAILY TARGETS, SO SERVE WITH 100G OF 0% FAT GREEK YOGHURT TO ADD 57 KCALS AND 10G OF PROTEIN. WE USE 0% GREEK YOGHURT AS THE GRANOLA ITSELF IS ALREADY HIGH IN FAT, THANKS TO THE NUTS AND SEEDS.

MAKES 8-10 SERVINGS

2 tablespoons coconut oil
6 tablespoons runny honey
1 teaspoon ground cinnamon
200g rolled oats
100g blanched almonds, halved
100g macadamia nuts, halved
50g flaxseed
50g pumpkin seeds
50g sunflower seeds
50g dried coconut flakes
100g raisins
100g dried cranberries

Preheat the oven to 160°C/gas mark 3.

Combine the coconut oil, honey and cinnamon in a pan and heat gently until the coconut oil has melted. Combine the remaining ingredients, except the raisins and cranberries, in a large bowl and pour over the oil and honey mixture. Stir to combine, making sure everything is evenly coated, then tip into a large non-stick roasting tin (if your tin isn't non-stick, line it with baking parchment first).

Bake for 20 minutes then remove from the oven and give everything a stir. Stir in the dried fruit and return to the oven for 10 minutes. Set aside to cool then pour into a large jar or airtight container.

USE IN THE FOLLOWING WAYS:

- Serve spooned over Greek yoghurt for breakfast
- Eat as cereal with almond milk and sliced banana
- Serve with the Cherry Choc Chip Frozen Yoghurt (see page 141)

PER SERVING: (based on 10 servings)
KCAL: 460   FAT: 28g
CARBS: 43g   PROTEIN: 9g

PROTEIN OATS

THIS IS OUR TAKE ON THE CLASSIC PORRIDGE. ALL THE USUAL SUSPECTS ARE IN THERE, PLENTY OF CARBS AND BERRIES TO TOP IT WITH SOME SWEETNESS, BUT THERE IS NOW A MUCH BIGGER PROTEIN KICK TO IT. USE WHATEVER FLAVOUR OF WHEY PROTEIN POWDER YOU PREFER – CHOCOLATE WOULD ALSO WORK WELL.

SERVES 1

40g rolled oats

1 scoop plain or vanilla whey protein
    powder (30g)

300ml coconut milk

Handful of fresh raspberries (60g),
    plus extra to serve

Stir the oats and protein powder together in a pan then pour in the coconut milk and raspberries. Slowly bring to a simmer then cook for 5 minutes until thickened, stirring occasionally.

Serve topped with a few fresh raspberries.

PER SERVING:
KCAL: 360   FAT: 12g
CARBS: 33g   PROTEIN: 29g

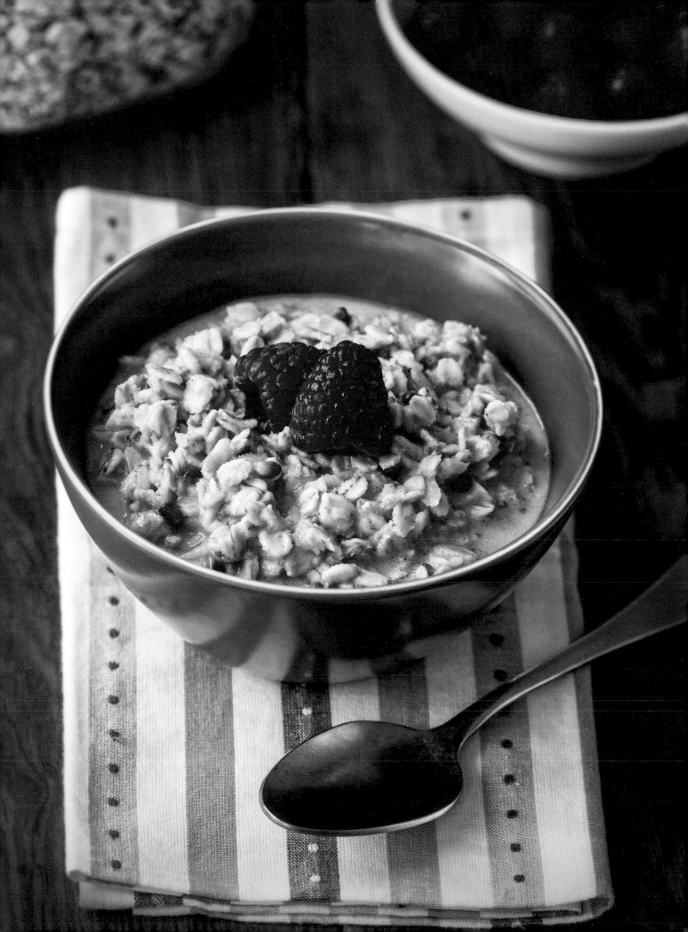

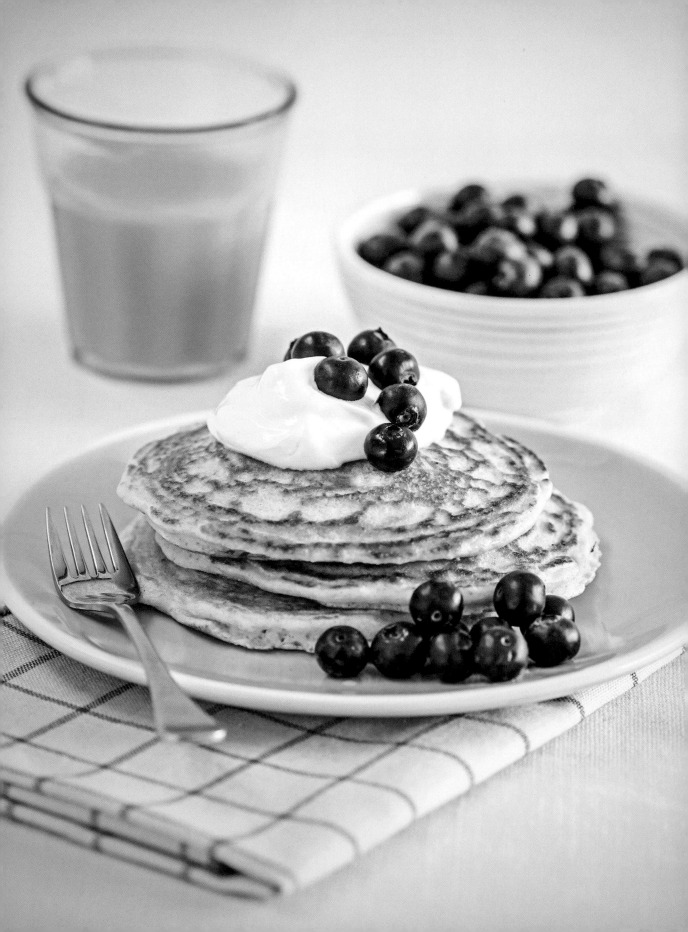

PROTEIN PANCAKES WITH BLUEBERRIES

THESE PANCAKES ARE GREAT FOR A MORNING TRAINING DAY BREAKFAST. THE POSSIBILITIES FOR DIFFERENT TOPPINGS ARE ENDLESS, SO BE AS CREATIVE AS YOU DARE. JUST REMEMBER THAT THE CALORIES AND MACRONUTRIENTS WILL BE AFFECTED BY ADDED INGREDIENTS.

MAKES 4

50g rolled oats
1 medium free-range egg
2 medium free-range egg whites
125ml unsweetened almond milk
1½ scoops vanilla whey protein
    powder (45g)
1 teaspoon baking powder
1 teaspoon coconut oil
2 tablespoons Greek yoghurt
Handful of blueberries (40g)

Simply grab a blender and pour in the oats, egg, egg whites, almond milk, protein powder and baking powder. Whizz until smooth.

Heat a non-stick frying pan and add the coconut oil. When it's hot, add a quarter of the pancake mixture to the centre of the pan and cook for 1–2 minutes. When you see bubbles rising on the surface, flip over and cook for a further 1–2 minutes until golden brown. Repeat with the remaining mixture and serve with the yoghurt and blueberries.

PER PANCAKE:
KCAL: 180   FAT: 7g
CARBS: 12g   PROTEIN: 17g

SUMMER FRUIT SALAD

THIS IS A LOVELY, LIGHT, CARB-RICH AND LOW-CALORIE START TO THE DAY. YOU MAY WANT TO ADD A SPRINKLE OF GROUND FLAXSEED ON TOP, OR MAYBE EVEN HAVE ONE OF OUR OATMEAL RAISIN COOKIES (SEE PAGE 149) WITH IT TO KEEP YOU GOING UNTIL LUNCH TIME.

SERVES 4

400g strawberries, hulled and halved

400g black grapes, halved

2 ripe peaches, stoned and sliced

300g raspberries

150g blueberries

TO SERVE

3 sprigs of mint, leaves torn

Put 100g of the strawberries into a food processor and blend until smooth. Combine the remaining ingredients in a large bowl, pour over the strawberry purée and toss to combine. Transfer to the fridge and chill for 1 hour.

Remove from the fridge, stir through the mint leaves and serve.

SERVING IDEAS:

- Serve with Greek yoghurt and a handful of Granola (see page 63)
- Blend any leftover salad to make a smoothie

PER SERVING:
KCAL: 176   FAT: 1g
CARBS: 43g   PROTEIN: 2g

POACHED EGGS ON TOAST WITH SPINACH

THIS IS A GOOD HEARTY BREAKFAST, GIVING A NICE KICK OF CARBS AND PROTEIN BUT NOT FORGETTING A GOOD PORTION OF HEALTHY FAT TOO. JUST REMEMBER TO FULLY DRY YOUR SPINACH BEFORE PUTTING IT ON THE TOAST – NOBODY LIKES SOGGY BREAD!

SERVES 1

2 medium free-range eggs
200g baby leaf spinach
1 thick slice of wholemeal toast
Sea salt and black pepper

Bring a large pan of unsalted water to a gentle simmer. Swirl the water gently and then crack the eggs in and poach for 3–4 minutes until the whites are just set.

Meanwhile heat a deep frying pan over a high heat, add a splash of water then throw in the spinach. Cook for 2 minutes until wilted then tip onto a clean tea towel. Wrap the spinach up tightly then squeeze out as much excess water as possible.

Lay the spinach on the toast, season with salt and pepper and top with the poached eggs.

PER SERVING:
KCAL: 282   FAT: 10g
CARBS: 22g   PROTEIN: 22g

SMASHED AVOCADO BAGELS WITH POACHED EGGS

THIS IS A BIG, FIRING-ON-ALL-CYLINDERS KINDA BREAKFAST, FULLY LOADED WITH GREAT STUFF, ALTHOUGH YOU CAN LEAVE OUT THE CREAM CHEESE IF YOU WANT TO KEEP YOUR CALORIES LOWER. THIS IS ONE OF OUR FAVOURITES TO PULL OUT ON THOSE REALLY ACHY TIRED DAYS WHEN WE'VE BEEN LOWER CARB FOR A FEW DAYS AND NEED BRINGING BACK TO LIFE. OH, AND IT TASTES GREAT TOO!

SERVES 2

2 medium free-range eggs

1 ripe medium avocado (150g)

Juice of 1 lime

1 red chilli, deseeded and
    finely chopped

Small bunch of coriander (25g),
    roughly chopped

Sea salt and black pepper

TO SERVE

1 seeded bagel

75g full-fat cream cheese* (optional)

Bring a large pan of unsalted water to a gentle simmer. Swirl the water gently and then crack the eggs in and poach for 3–4 minutes until the whites are just set.

Meanwhile halve the avocado and scoop the flesh into a bowl. Add the lime juice, chilli and coriander and roughly smash with a fork; keep it nice and chunky. Season.

Toast the bagel, spread each half with cream cheese (if using) then spoon over the smashed avocado. Top with the poached eggs and serve.

PER SERVING: (*without cream cheese)
KCAL: 460 (*360)   FAT: 26g (*17g)
CARBS: 40g (*39g)   PROTEIN: 16g (*14g)

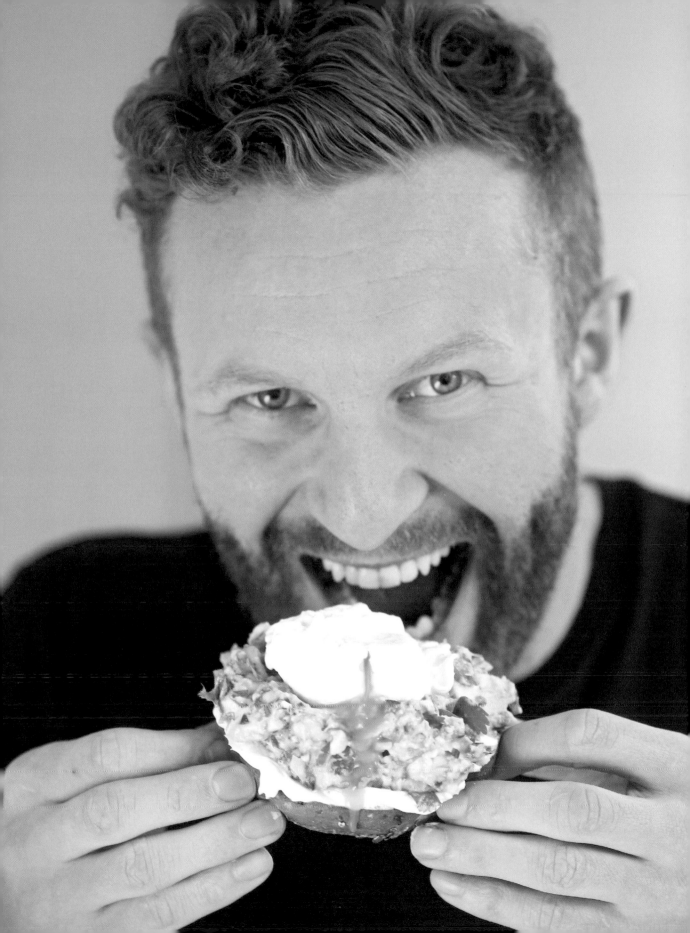

SALMON WITH AVOCADO

BY FAR ONE OF OUR FAVOURITE BREAKFASTS TO COOK UP, THIS COVERS ALL BASES, TAKES HARDLY ANY TIME TO MAKE AND TASTES GREAT. IF YOU'RE ON A LOWER-CARB DAY SIMPLY TAKE AWAY THE WHOLEMEAL BREAD AND SERVE THE MASHED AVOCADO ALONGSIDE THE SALMON – JUST AS DELICIOUS.

SERVES 1

2 teaspoons coconut oil

150g salmon fillet, skin on

Sea salt and black pepper

1 ripe medium avocado (150g)

Juice of ½ lemon, plus a lemon
   wedge to serve

1 slice of wholemeal bread*

Heat the coconut oil in a frying pan over a medium heat. Score the salmon skin with a sharp knife, season with salt and pepper then lay in the pan skin-side down. Fry for 4–5 minutes, shaking the pan, then turn and cook for a further 2 minutes.

Meanwhile halve the avocado, scoop the flesh into a bowl and add the lemon juice. Roughly mash together with a fork and season to taste.

Toast the bread, top with the avocado and salmon and serve with a lemon wedge.

PER SERVING: (*without bread)
KCAL: 628 (*575)   FAT: 48g (*47g)
CARBS: 14g (*5g)   PROTEIN: 35g (*33g)

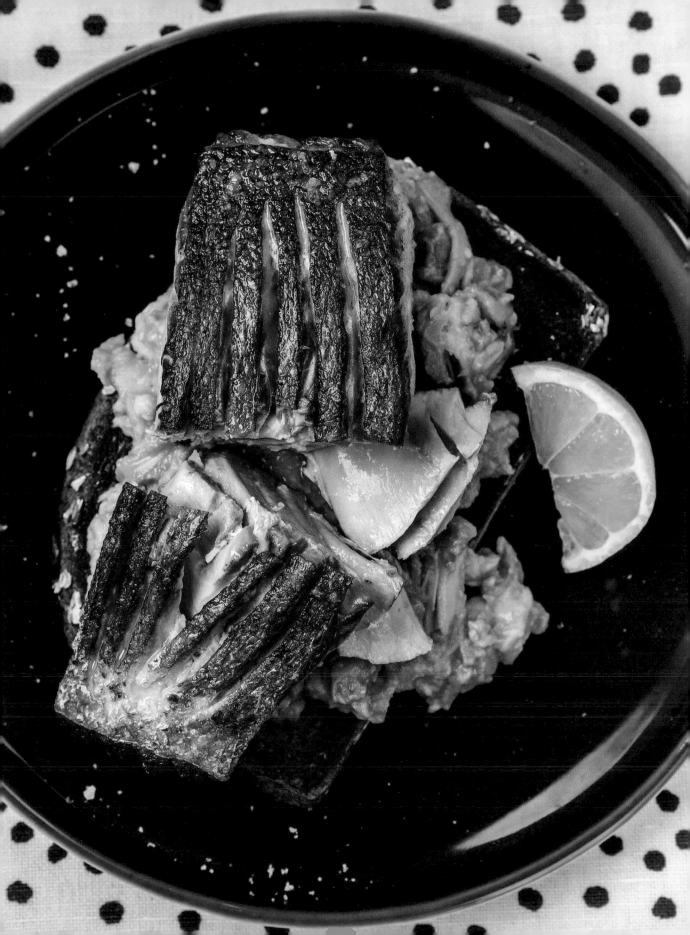

KEDGEREE

IF YOU'VE NOT TRIED THIS BEFORE, IT'S A MUST! SMOKY AND SPICY, IT'S A GREAT WAY OF GETTING MORE FISH INTO YOUR DIET. IT ALSO GIVES YOU A DOUBLE PROTEIN HIT FROM THE EGGS, TO GET YOU FEELING TOTALLY READY FOR YOUR MORNING WORKOUT.

SERVES 2

300ml milk
1 bay leaf
240g undyed smoked haddock
2 medium free-range eggs
1 tablespoon coconut oil
1 small onion, finely chopped
2 teaspoons curry powder
1 x 250g pouch cooked basmati rice
Small bunch of parsley (25g), chopped
Lemon wedges, to serve

Pour the milk into a pan, add the bay leaf and bring to a gentle simmer. Lower the haddock into the milk and poach for 5–6 minutes until the fish flakes easily. Remove from the pan with a slotted spoon (reserving the milk for later) and set aside until cool enough to handle.

Meanwhile boil the eggs for 5 minutes, drain and run under cold water to stop them from cooking further. Peel the shells away and cut the eggs in half.

Heat the coconut oil in a deep frying pan, add the onion and fry for 5 minutes until soft. Add the curry powder and fry for a minute. Stir in the rice and 3 tablespoons of the milk from the fish pan and cook for a couple of minutes to warm through. Flake the fish, discarding the skin and any bones then stir through the rice.

Divide between two serving bowls, top with the egg halves and sprinkle over the parsley. Serve with the lemon wedges.

PER SERVING:
KCAL: 485   FAT: 17g
CARBS: 41g   PROTEIN: 41g

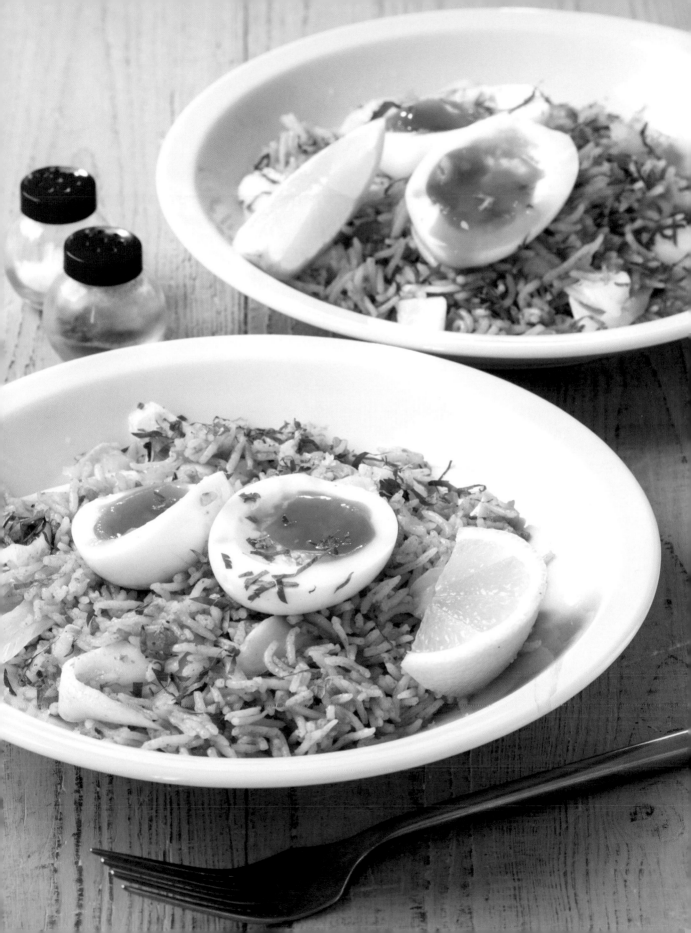

BREAKFAST BURRITOS

NOW THIS IS ONE HELL OF A CALORIFIC START TO THE DAY, GETTING YOU READY TO FACE THE GRIND – AND THEN SOME. ONE THING THAT A LOT OF PEOPLE FORGET ABOUT BURRITOS IS THAT THE FILLING ITSELF MAKES FOR A FANTASTIC STIR-FRY IF YOU ARE WATCHING YOUR CARB INTAKE. JUST LEAVING OUT THE TORTILLA WRAPS WILL SAVE YOU A GOOD 34G CARBS AND 200 CALORIES PER SERVING.

SERVES 2

2 large field mushrooms, stalks
    removed (130g)
8 cherry tomatoes, halved
Sea salt and black pepper
4 rashers smoked back bacon
    (150g), fat trimmed
1 x 400g tin black beans,
    rinsed and drained
Pinch of chilli flakes
1 tablespoon olive oil
4 medium free-range eggs, beaten
2 large flour tortillas
50g mature Cheddar, grated
Chilli sauce, to serve

Preheat the grill to high. Lay the mushrooms and tomatoes on a baking tray, season with salt and pepper then lay the bacon alongside. Grill for 6–7 minutes, turning the mushrooms and bacon halfway through. Remove from the grill and thinly slice the mushrooms.

Meanwhile put the black beans in a pan with the chilli flakes and a splash of water and heat gently for 5 minutes until softened. Roughly mash with a fork.

Heat the oil in a separate pan, add the eggs and cook gently for 3–4 minutes, stirring all the time, until scrambled.

To serve, heat the tortillas in a microwave for 30 seconds (or for a few minutes in a low oven) until soft. Spread with the black beans and sprinkle over the cheese. Top with the scrambled eggs, sliced mushrooms, the bacon and tomatoes. Fold the sides in then roll up tightly. Serve with chilli sauce.

PER SERVING:
KCAL: 593   FAT: 32g
CARBS: 41g   PROTEIN: 38g

SWEET POTATO HASH BROWNS

THERE'S NO MESSING AROUND HERE: BACON, EGGS AND SWEET POTATO FOR BREAKFAST AND FOR ONLY 556 CALORIES PER SERVING. COOKED IN COCONUT OIL, WITH ITS HIGH SMOKE POINT, THIS IS A MUCH-HEALTHIER VERSION OF YOUR REGULAR FRY-UP. FOR US THIS IS AN IDEAL SUNDAY MORNING BREAKFAST WHEN WE HAVE A BIT MORE TIME TO PREP; WE CAN THEN HEAD TO THE GYM FEELING WELL FUELLED.

SERVES 2

400g sweet potato

1 x 400g tin red kidney beans, rinsed and drained

4 spring onions, finely chopped

2 tablespoons sundried tomato and herb paste

1 tablespoon coconut oil

Sea salt and black pepper

TO SERVE

1 teaspoon coconut oil

4 rashers back bacon, fat trimmed

2 medium free-range eggs

Pierce the sweet potatoes a couple of times with a skewer or sharp knife then microwave for 10 minutes, or until soft. (Alternatively bake in a 200°C/gas mark 6 oven for about 45 minutes.) Leave to cool slightly then cut in half and scoop the flesh into a mixing bowl. Add the kidney beans, spring onions, and tomato and herb paste then roughly mash with a potato masher. Season to taste then shape into four rounds.

Heat the coconut oil in a frying pan over a medium heat, add the hash browns and fry for 3–4 minutes on each side.

Meanwhile fry the bacon in a separate frying pan for 2 minutes, then turn over. Crack the eggs into the pan and cook everything for a couple of minutes, until the eggs are cooked to your liking. Serve the hash browns with the bacon and eggs.

PER SERVING:
KCAL: 556   FAT: 24g
CARBS: 52g   PROTEIN: 33g

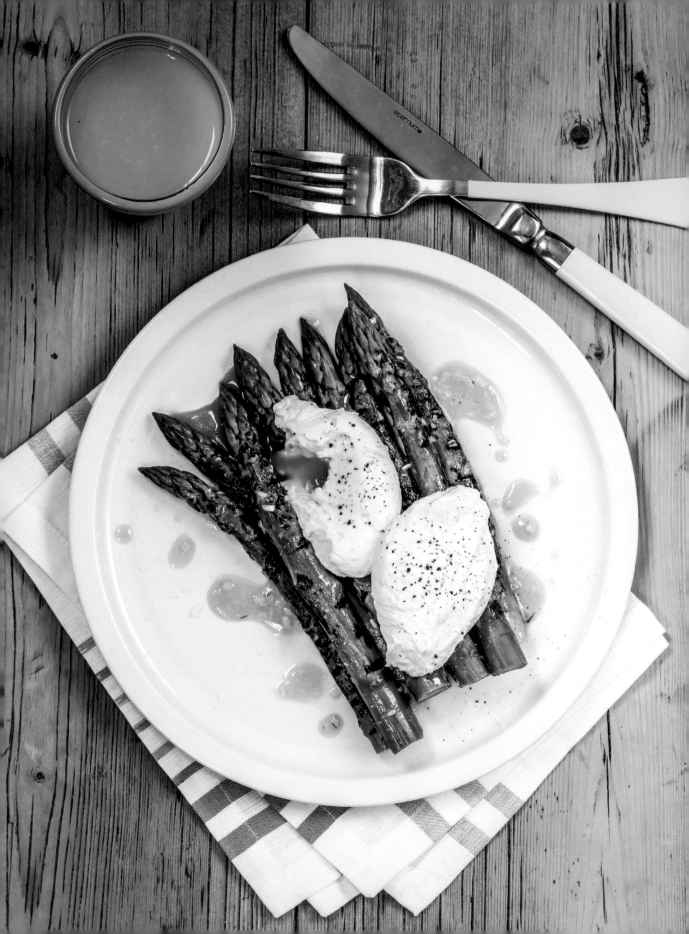

GRILLED ASPARAGUS WITH POACHED EGGS

A REAL LOW-CARB OPTION AND A GREAT BREAKFAST FOR THOSE OF US WHO FEEL BETTER EATING FEWER CARBS AND MORE FAT AND PROTEIN IN THE MORNING. THIS IS AN IDEAL MEAL FOR THOSE OF US WHOSE JOBS ARE LESS ACTIVE AND POTENTIALLY FOR NON-TRAINING DAYS. REDUCING YOUR CARBS AND CALORIES ON THESE DAYS CAN HELP YOU STAY LEAN AND IMPROVE YOUR ABILITY TO SWITCH BETWEEN USING FAT AND CARBS AS A PRIMARY ENERGY SOURCE, KNOWN AS METABOLIC FLEXIBILITY (SEE PAGE 47 FOR MORE ON THIS).

SERVES 2

2 x 300g bunches of asparagus
4 medium free-range eggs

FOR THE DRESSING

1 shallot, finely chopped
2 tablespoons extra-virgin olive oil
1 tablespoon white wine vinegar
1 teaspoon Dijon mustard
Sea salt and black pepper

To prepare the asparagus, bend each steam near the base until it snaps; discard the woody ends. Bring a large pan of salted water to the boil and blanch the asparagus for 2 minutes. Drain and pat dry on kitchen paper.

Whisk together the ingredients for the dressing in a large bowl and season to taste.

Bring a large pan of unsalted water to a gentle simmer. Swirl the water gently and then crack the eggs in and poach for 3–4 minutes until the whites are just set.

While the eggs are cooking, heat a heavy griddle pan over a high heat then griddle the asparagus for 3–4 minutes, turning regularly, until lightly charred. Transfer to the bowl of dressing and toss to coat. Pile the asparagus onto a plate, top with the poached eggs and serve.

PER SERVING:
KCAL: 330   FAT: 22g
CARBS: 12g   PROTEIN: 21g

LENTIL, BEETROOT +
GOATS' CHEESE SALAD

EVERYBODY LOVES A SALAD – THIS IS OUR TASTY LITTLE NUMBER. IT'S ALL TOO EASY TO BE BORING AND JUST CHUCK A FEW LEAVES ON A PLATE. A LITTLE EXTRA PREP OF BAKING THE PEPPERS REALLY TAKES THIS SIMPLE SALAD TO THE NEXT LEVEL.

SERVES 2

2 medium red peppers

1 x 250g pouch cooked lentils

3 cooked beetroot (200g), cut into wedges

2 tablespoons olive oil

1 tablespoon sherry vinegar or red wine vinegar

2 teaspoons Dijon mustard

Sea salt and black pepper

75g goats' cheese, crumbled

70g bag rocket leaves

Preheat the oven to 220°C/gas mark 7. Lay the peppers on a baking tray and roast for 20 minutes, turning halfway through cooking. Transfer to a bowl, cover with cling film and leave to steam and cool. After 10 minutes peel the peppers, discard the stalk and seeds and tear the flesh into strips.

Reheat the lentils according to the packet instructions then pour into a large bowl and combine with the peppers and beetroot.

In a separate bowl, whisk together the oil, vinegar and mustard, season to taste then pour over the lentils. Add the goats' cheese and rocket and gently toss to combine.

PER SERVING:
KCAL: 483   FAT: 27g
CARBS: 39g   PROTEIN: 21g

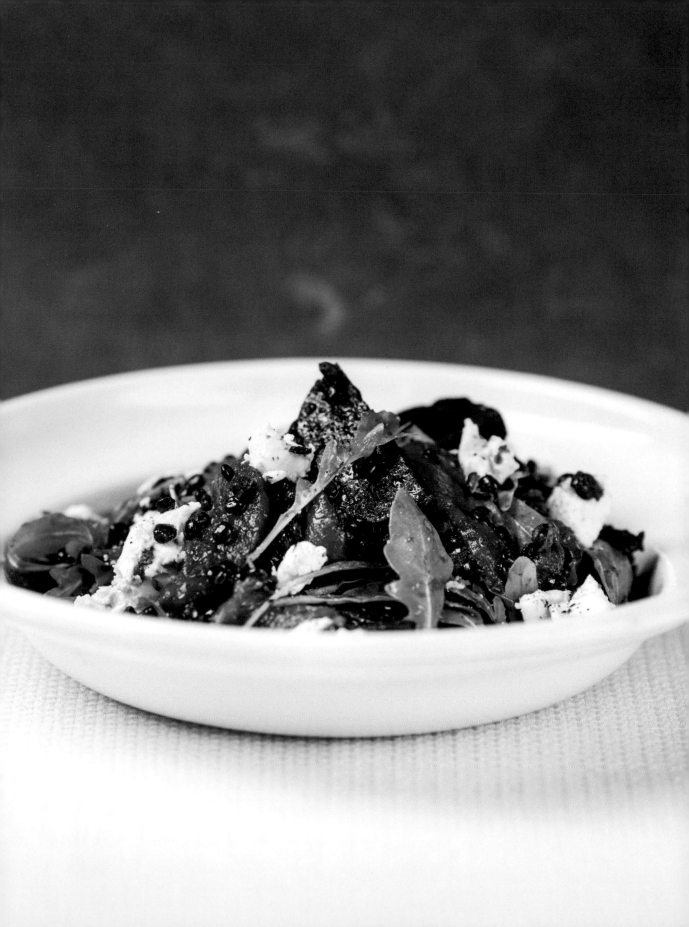

QUICK BEAN CHILLI WITH CHIPOTLE

THIS QUICK BEAN CHILLI IS AN INCREDIBLE VARIATION ON THE NORMAL CHILLI SET-UP AND GIVES YOU SO MANY OPTIONS. YOU CAN SERVE IT WITH RICE, BAKED SWEET POTATOES OR EVEN FLOUR WRAPS – WHATEVER TAKES YOUR FANCY. THE MACRONUTRIENT/CALORIE SPLIT IS FOR SERVING WITHOUT RICE OR SWEET POTATOES SO REMEMBER THAT THE NUMBERS WILL BE AFFECTED, DEPENDING ON HOW YOU CHOOSE TO SERVE THE CHILLI.

SERVES 4

1 tablespoon olive oil
2 medium onions, finely chopped
2 garlic cloves, crushed
2 red chillies, deseeded and
    finely chopped
2 teaspoons ground cumin
1 tablespoon tomato purée
2 teaspoons chipotle chilli paste
1 x 400g tin chopped tomatoes
2 x 400g tins mixed beans,
    rinsed and drained
150ml vegetable stock
Sea salt and black pepper

TO SERVE

150ml soured cream
Small bunch of coriander (25g),
    chopped

Heat the oil in a large, heavy-based pan and add the onions. Fry gently for 5 minutes until softened, add the garlic and chilli and fry for a further 2 minutes. Stir in the ground cumin then add the tomato purée and chipotle paste. Cook for a minute then add the tomatoes, beans and stock. Simmer gently for 15 minutes until thickened, then remove from the heat and season to taste.

Serve the chilli with rice or baked sweet potatoes and top with a spoonful of soured cream and some chopped coriander.

PER SERVING:
KCAL: 231   FAT: 7g
CARBS: 38g   PROTEIN: 4g

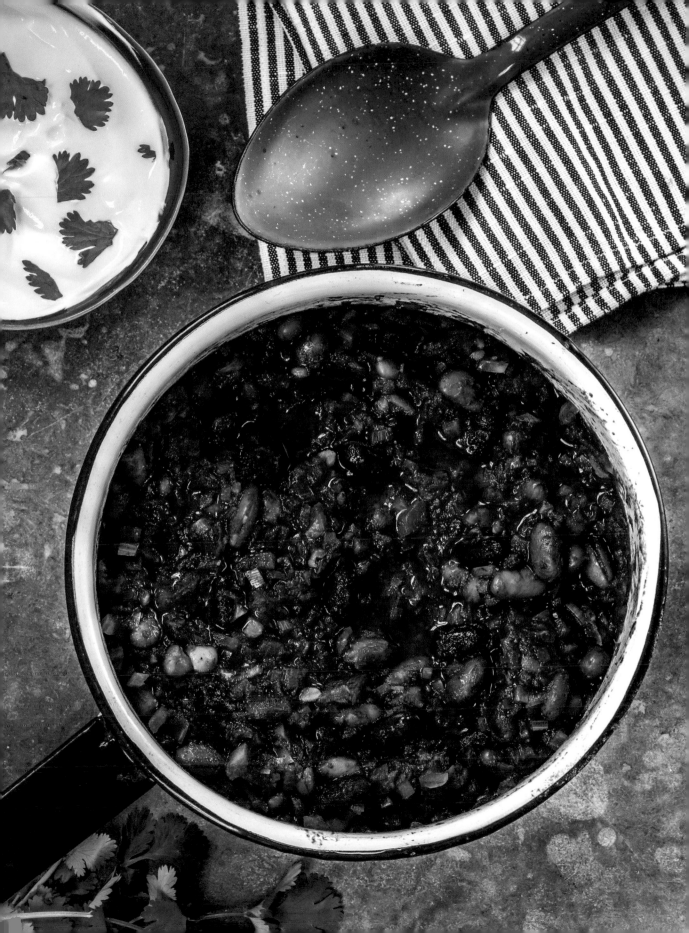

LOADED SWEET POTATO SKINS

THIS IS A SUPER TASTY MEAL BUT QUITE LIKELY TO USE A LOT OF YOUR DAILY FAT INTAKE, SO IF YOU WANT TO SAVE CALORIES, SWAP THE FULL-FAT CREAM CHEESE FOR A REDUCED-FAT OR LIGHT OPTION.

SERVES 2

2 medium sweet potatoes
   (350g each)
1 tablespoon olive oil
4 rashers unsmoked back bacon
   (140g), fat trimmed, chopped
1 small onion, finely chopped
1 garlic clove, crushed
200g baby leaf spinach
50g full-fat cream cheese
Sea salt and black pepper
75g mozzarella or mature Cheddar,
   grated

Preheat the oven to 200°C/gas mark 6.

Pierce the sweet potatoes a couple of times with a skewer or sharp knife then microwave for 15 minutes, or until soft, then set aside to cool. (Alternatively bake in a 200°C/gas mark 6 oven for about 45 minutes.)

Meanwhile heat the oil in a frying pan, add the bacon and fry for 3–4 minutes until crisp. Remove from the pan with a slotted spoon and set aside. Add the onion to the pan, fry for 5 minutes until soft then add the garlic. Fry for a minute then increase the heat and add the spinach. Cook for a couple of minutes until wilted then remove from the heat and tip into a bowl. Stir in the bacon and cream cheese.

Cut the sweet potatoes in half and scoop the flesh into the bowl. Stir to combine and season to taste. Lay the empty sweet potato skins on a baking tray and cook in the oven for 5 minutes until crisp.

Spoon the filling into the skins, top with the mozzarella or Cheddar and bake for 10 minutes until the cheese has melted.

PER SERVING:
KCAL: 696   FAT: 32g
CARBS: 74g   PROTEIN: 28g

SALMON + BLACK BEAN SALAD

AS WELL AS TASTING DELICIOUS, SALMON IS A GREAT WAY TO GET SOME HEALTHY FATS INTO YOUR DIET. ADD SOME BLACK BEANS AND YOU WILL BE CREATING A GREAT HIGH-PROTEIN MEAL, MAKING THIS IDEAL POST-WORKOUT.

SERVES 1

2 teaspoons coconut oil

150g salmon fillet, skin on

Sea salt and black pepper

½ x 400g tin black beans, rinsed and drained

6 cherry tomatoes, halved

½ cucumber, sliced

1 baby gem lettuce, leaves torn

Handful of croutons (20g)

1 tablespoon sweet chilli sauce

Heat the coconut oil in a frying pan over a medium heat. Score the salmon skin with a sharp knife, season with salt and pepper then lay in the pan skin-side down. Fry for 4–5 minutes moving the fish or shaking then pan, then turn and cook for a further 2 minutes.

Meanwhile combine the beans, tomatoes, cucumber, lettuce and croutons in a large bowl. Pour over the sweet chilli sauce, toss to combine and serve with the salmon.

PER SERVING:
KCAL: 682   FAT: 38g
CARBS: 37g   PROTEIN: 47g

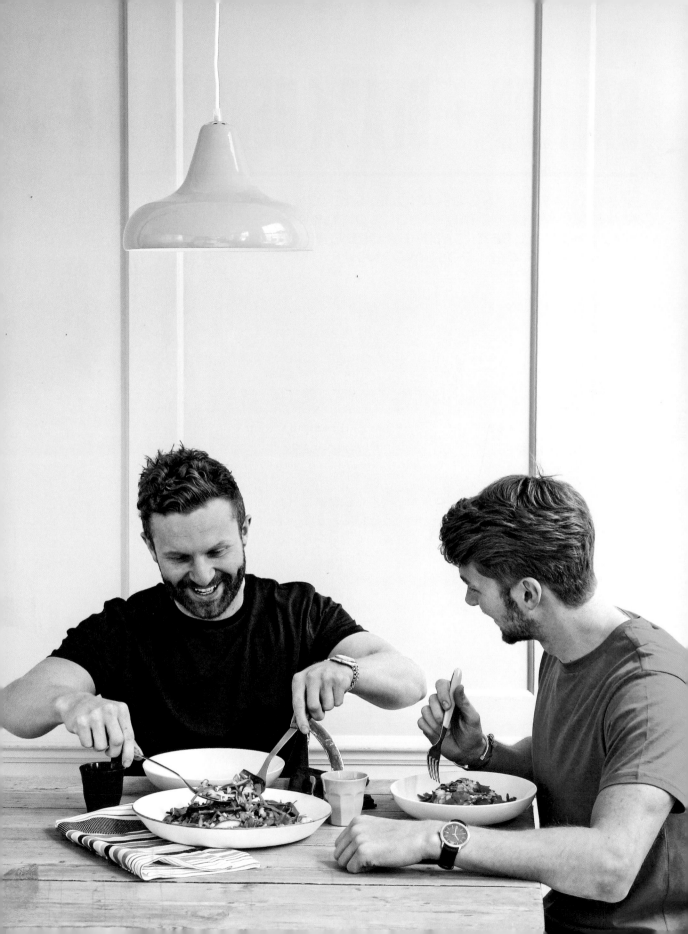

THAI PRAWN SALAD

THIS IS A GREAT SALAD FOR A LOWER-CARB REST DAY LUNCH OR EVEN ON A TRAINING DAY. IF YOU HAVE ALREADY TRAINED AND WANT TO BOOST YOUR CARBS, SIMPLY SERVE WITH 300G COOKED RICE TO HELP THAT RECOVERY AND REPLENISHMENT OF YOUR MUSCLE STORES.

SERVES 2

300g cooked, peeled tiger prawns

2 medium carrots, cut into matchsticks

1 medium red pepper, deseeded and finely sliced

½ cucumber, halved, deseeded and finely sliced

4 spring onions, finely sliced

100g green beans, sliced

2 tablespoon roasted peanuts, crushed

Small bunch of coriander (25g), leaves roughly torn

FOR THE DRESSING*

2 tablespoons fish sauce

Juice of 1 lime

2 teaspoons palm sugar

1 garlic clove, crushed

1 red bird's eye chilli, deseeded and finely chopped

Combine all of the salad ingredients in a large bowl.

For the dressing, whisk the fish sauce, lime juice and palm sugar together in a separate bowl until the sugar has dissolved, then whisk in the garlic and chilli. Pour over the salad, toss to combine and serve.

PER SERVING: (*without dressing)
KCAL: 330 (*250)   FAT: 8g (*8g)
CARBS: 35g (*18g)   PROTEIN: 32g (*30g)

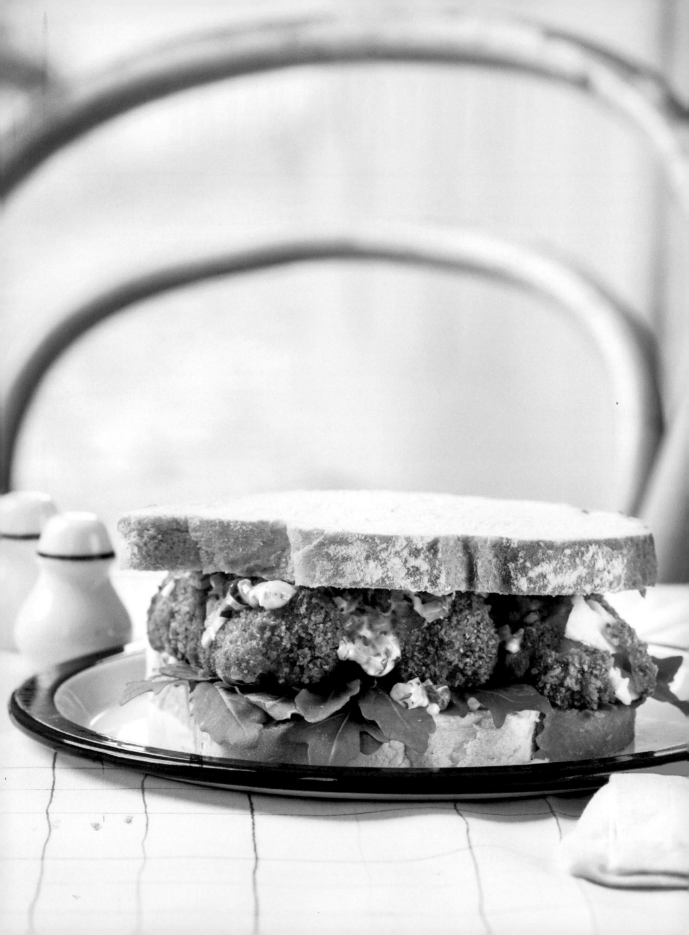

FISH FINGER SANDWICHES WITH TARTARE SAUCE

KEEP THIS MEAL FOR POST WORKOUT, OR FOR WHEN YOU HAVE A FEW CALORIES TO SPARE, AS IT'S RELATIVELY HIGH IN CALORIES AND CARBS. TO REDUCE THE CARBS AND SAVE ON CALORIES, SWAP THE BREAD FOR 160G GREEN SALAD.

SERVES 2

50g plain flour

300g cod fillet, cut into 6 equal fingers

2 medium free-range eggs, beaten

75g dry white breadcrumbs

½ teaspoon smoked paprika

Olive oil spray

Sea salt and black pepper

FOR THE TARTARE SAUCE

3 tablespoons mayonnaise

2 gherkins (30g), finely chopped

1 small shallot, finely chopped

1 tablespoon capers

Small bunch of parsley (25g),
   finely chopped

Lemon juice, to taste

TO SERVE

4 slices of white bread

Handful of rocket leaves (50g)

Preheat the oven to 180°C/gas mark 4 and line a baking tray with baking parchment.

Pour the flour into a sandwich bag and season with plenty of salt and pepper. Add the fish pieces, seal the bag and give it a good shake to coat the fish. Pour the beaten egg into a shallow dish and combine the breadcrumbs and paprika in a separate dish.

Coat the floured fish pieces in the beaten egg and then in the breadcrumbs. Repeat with the egg and breadcrumbs so that each piece of fish has had a double coating. Lay the fish fingers on the lined baking tray and spray with a little olive oil. Bake for 15 minutes until the fish is cooked through.

Meanwhile combine the ingredients for the tartare sauce in a bowl and add lemon juice to taste. Spread two slices of bread with the tartare sauce, top with the fish fingers and rocket, then sandwich with the remaining bread.

PER SERVING: (*with salad instead of bread)
KCAL: 670 (*543)   **FAT: 26g (*25g)**
CARBS: 74g (*49g)   **PROTEIN: 35g (*32g)**

SPICY CHICKEN WITH ROAST VEGETABLES

THIS IS ONE OF OUR FAVOURITE MEALS TO PUT TOGETHER ON A SUNDAY NIGHT AS IT TAKES VERY LITTLE TIME TO PREPARE AND IS EASY TO PUT TOGETHER. YOU CAN USE ANY OTHER VEG YOU HAVE TO HAND; IF YOU WANT TO MAKE IT A SLIGHTLY LOWER-CARB MEAL, JUST REDUCE THE AMOUNT OF SWEET POTATO.

SERVES 2

1 tablespoon olive oil

2 garlic cloves, crushed

1 teaspoon cayenne pepper

1 teaspoon ground cumin

Pinch of sea salt

2 medium sweet potatoes, peeled and cut into 2cm chunks (500g prepared weight)

1 small red onion, cut into wedges

1 courgette (160g), cut into 2cm chunks

2 large tomatoes, cut into wedges

1 medium yellow pepper, deseeded and cut into 2cm chunks

2 x 170g skinless chicken breasts, cut into bite-sized pieces

Preheat the oven to 200°C/gas mark 6.

Whisk together the oil, garlic, spices and salt in a large bowl, add the vegetables and toss to combine. Tip into a large roasting tin and roast for 35 minutes until the sweet potatoes are tender when pierced with a knife.

Add the chicken to the bowl used for the vegetables and toss to coat in the remaining spice mix.

Heat oil in a large frying pan or wok over a high heat, add the chicken and fry for 5–6 minutes until cooked through. Add the chicken to the vegetables, toss to combine and serve.

PER SERVING:
KCAL: 470 FAT: 2g
CARBS: 67g PROTEIN: 46g

CHICKEN, SWEETCORN + MUSHROOM SOUP

THIS SOUP IS GREAT IF YOU ARE LOOKING TO HIT YOUR PROTEIN TARGETS BUT KEEP YOUR TOTAL CALORIES DOWN, WHICH IS IMPORTANT WHEN DIETING. REMEMBER, IF YOU ARE IN A CALORIC DEFICIT TO LOSE FAT BUT YOUR PROTEIN IS VERY LOW YOU STAND A GOOD CHANCE OF LOSING IMPORTANT MUSCLE TOO! MUSCLE IS METABOLICALLY ACTIVE TISSUE, MEANING IT USES ENERGY AND BURNS FAT, MAKING DIETING EASIER.

SERVES 2

800ml fresh chicken stock

2 x 170g skinless chicken breasts

1 x 340g tin sweetcorn, drained

125g chestnut mushrooms, finely sliced

4 spring onions, finely sliced

Sea salt and black pepper

Pour the chicken stock into a pan and bring to the boil. Add the chicken breasts then reduce the heat to a simmer and poach for 8–10 minutes until cooked through. Remove from the pan and set aside to cool.

Add the sweetcorn to the pan, heat through for a couple of minutes then use a stick blender or liquidiser to roughly blend the soup. If you're using a liquidiser, blend half of the stock and sweetcorn and return it to the pan to keep some texture. Add the mushrooms and cook for 3–4 minutes until softened.

Using two forks, shred the poached chicken and then return it to the pan. Add the spring onions, heat through for a minute then season to taste and serve.

PER SERVING:
KCAL: 391   FAT: 9g
CARBS: 15g   PROTEIN: 60g

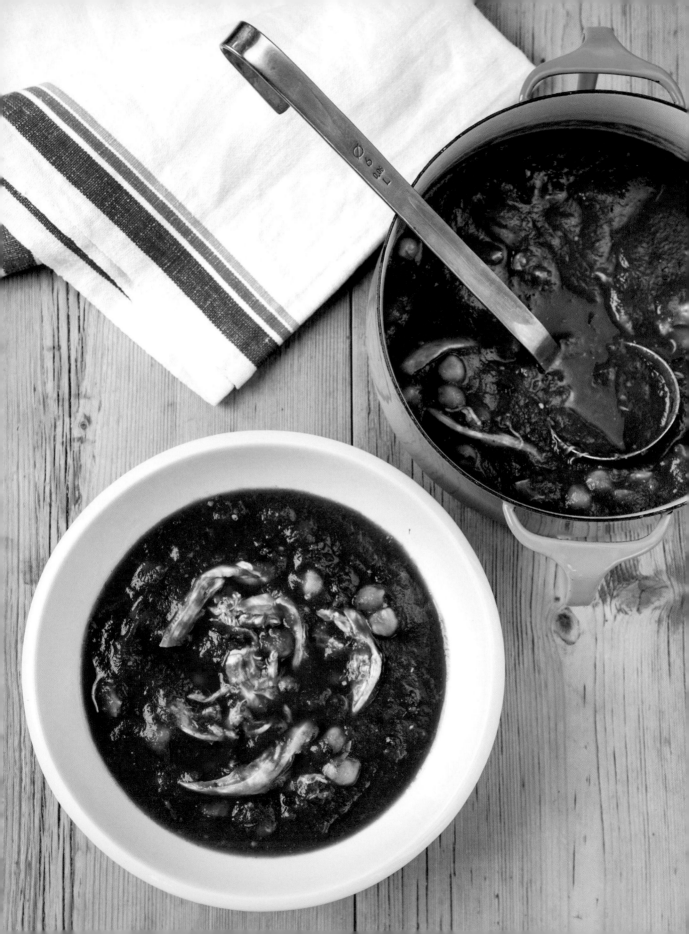

ROAST TOMATO, CHICKEN AND CHICKPEA SOUP

SOUPS ARE SUPER-EASY TO PREPARE AHEAD OF TIME; MAKE UP A DOUBLE BATCH AND KEEP IN THE FRIDGE OR EVEN FREEZE PORTIONS FOR LATER. THEY MAKE A GREAT LOWER-CARB MEAL TOO.

SERVES 2

500g ripe tomatoes, halved

1 small red onion, cut into wedges

2 garlic cloves, unpeeled

750ml fresh chicken stock

2 x 150g skinless chicken breasts

2 tablespoons tomato purée

Small bunch of basil (20g),
   leaves torn

1 x 400g tin chickpeas,
   rinsed and drained

Sea salt and black pepper

Preheat the oven to 220°C/gas mark 7. Lay the tomatoes, onion and garlic on a baking tray and roast for 20 minutes.

Meanwhile pour the chicken stock into a pan and bring to the boil. Add the chicken breasts then reduce the heat to a simmer and poach for 8–10 minutes until cooked through. Remove from the pan and set aside to cool.

Remove the tomatoes from the oven, peel the garlic and add everything to the pan of stock. Stir in the tomato purée and simmer for 2 minutes. Stir in the basil then use a stick blender or liquidiser to blend the soup until smooth.

Add the chickpeas and reheat for a couple of minutes. Using two forks, shred the poached chicken and add to the soup. Season to taste and serve.

PER SERVING:
KCAL: 430   FAT: 9g
CARBS: 37g   PROTEIN: 51g

JERK CHICKEN WRAPS WITH PINEAPPLE SALSA

THIS IS A GREAT HIGH-PROTEIN MEAL, BUT WITH A GOOD AMOUNT OF FAT AND CARBS TOO. THESE TYPES OF MEALS ARE GREAT TO PUT INTO YOUR DIET PLAN AS THEY ARE RELATIVELY BALANCED IN TERMS OF MACRONUTRIENTS. EATING MEALS THAT ARE SUPER-HIGH IN JUST ONE MACRONUTRIENT OFTEN MAKES IT HARD TO STICK TO YOUR DAILY TARGETS.

SERVES 2

2 teaspoons coconut oil, melted

2 teaspoons jerk seasoning

2 x 150g skinless chicken breasts, butterflied

FOR THE PINEAPPLE SALSA

½ small pineapple (125g), peeled, cored and finely chopped

1 small red onion, finely chopped

1 red chilli, deseeded and finely chopped

1 ripe tomato, deseeded and finely chopped

Small bunch of coriander (25g), chopped

Juice of 1 lime

Sea salt and black pepper

TO SERVE

2 large tortilla wraps

1 baby gem lettuce, leaves separated

Preheat a griddle pan to a high heat. Combine the coconut oil and jerk seasoning in a large bowl, add the chicken breasts and toss to coat. Griddle the chicken for 3–4 minutes on each side until cooked through then set aside to rest for 5 minutes.

Meanwhile combine the ingredients for the salsa in a bowl and season to taste.

Toss the lettuce leaves on the tortilla, slice the chicken into strips and place on top, then spoon over the salsa. Wrap up and enjoy.

PER SERVING:
KCAL: 484   FAT: 16g
CARBS: 43g   PROTEIN: 39g

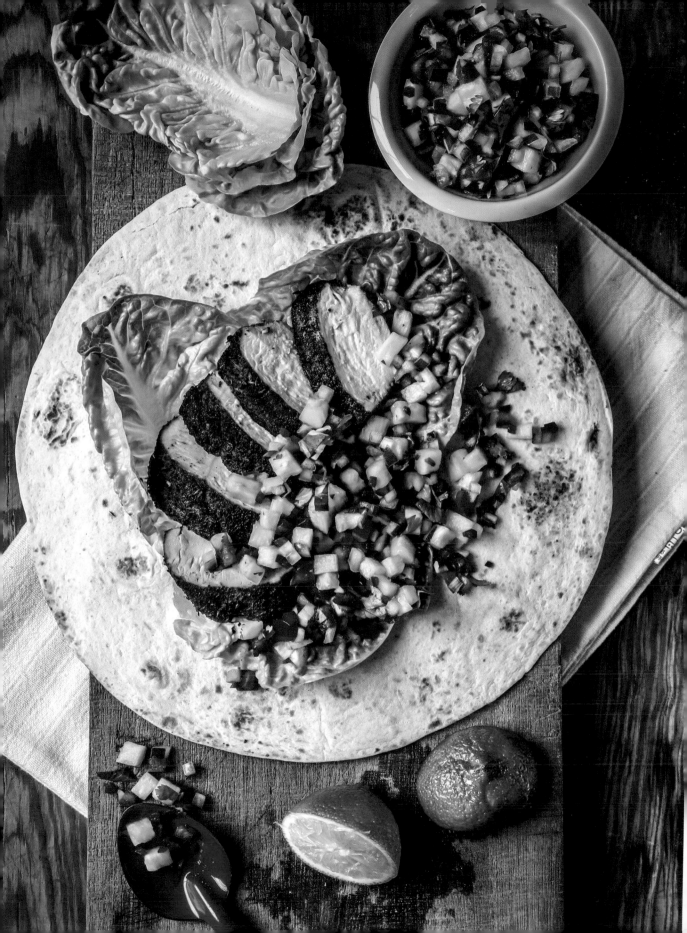

CHICKEN WITH FETA + BACON

THIS IS SUCH A GREAT WAY TO TAKE YOUR AVERAGE CHICKEN BREAST TO AN AWESOME LEVEL IN ONE SIMPLE STEP. IT TASTES AMAZING BUT IF YOU WANT TO REDUCE THE AMOUNT OF FAT, SIMPLY LEAVE OUT THE BACON. YOU COULD ALSO USE A LOWER-FAT CHEESE INSTEAD OF THE FETA.

SERVES 2

2 x 170g skinless chicken breasts

100g feta cheese, crumbled

4 rashers unsmoked back bacon (150g), fat trimmed

1 tablespoon coconut oil

1 medium red pepper, deseeded and thinly sliced

1 medium green pepper, deseeded and thinly sliced

1 red chilli, deseeded and finely chopped

1 garlic clove, crushed

½ teaspoon cayenne pepper

Sea salt and black pepper

Preheat the oven to 180°C/gas mark 4 and line a baking tray with foil or baking parchment.

Using a small, sharp knife, make a small slit in the side of each chicken breast then move the tip of the knife from side to side to make a pocket. Stuff half of the feta into each breast then wrap each in two slices of bacon. Lay the chicken on the baking tray and cook in the oven for 25 minutes.

While the chicken is cooking, heat the oil in a frying pan, add the peppers and fry gently for 5 minutes until soft. Add the chilli, garlic and cayenne pepper and cook for a further 1–2 minutes, then add a splash of water and season to taste.

Remove the chicken from the oven and set aside to rest for 5 minutes before serving with the peppers.

PER SERVING:
KCAL: 540   FAT: 29g
CARBS: 8g   PROTEIN: 60g

STEAK + PEPPER WRAPS

THIS COMBINES TWO THINGS THAT WE ABSOLUTELY LOVE: STEAK AND WRAPS! WRAPS ARE SO SIMPLE TO PREPARE AND MAKE A GREAT DISH TO SHARE WITH FRIENDS, SO DOUBLE THE QUANTITIES HERE FOR A SOCIABLE MEAL WITH FRIENDS – SIMPLY PUT THE WRAPS, FILLING AND LETTUCE IN THE MIDDLE OF THE TABLE AND LET EVERYONE GET STUCK IN. AND, IF YOU FANCY A CHANGE OF PROTEIN, WHY NOT USE CHICKEN BREAST INSTEAD? IF YOU'RE LOOKING TO REDUCE YOUR CARB INTAKE, SIMPLY ENJOY THE FILLING WITHOUT THE WRAPS.

SERVES 2

1 tablespoon coconut oil

1 fillet steak, around 170–200g, sliced into 2cm thick strips

1 medium red pepper, deseeded and finely sliced

1 medium green pepper, deseeded and finely sliced

1 red chilli, deseeded and finely chopped

6 chestnut mushrooms, thinly sliced

2 large tortilla wraps* or Protein Flatbreads (see page 105)

1 baby gem lettuce, leaves separated

Sea salt and black pepper

Heat half of the coconut oil in a large frying pan over a high heat. Add the steak strips and fry for 2–3 minutes until browned. Remove from the pan with a slotted spoon and set aside.

Heat the remaining oil in the pan, add the peppers, chilli and mushrooms and fry for 3–4 minutes until softened. Return the beef to the pan, toss everything together and season to taste. Divide the beef and vegetables between the two wraps, top with the lettuces leaves and wrap up tightly.

PER SERVING: (*without wrap)
KCAL: 420 (*240)   FAT: 14g (*10g)
CARBS: 38g (*7g)   PROTEIN: 35g (*30g)

QUICK STEAK TACOS WITH GUACAMOLE

OKAY, SO THIS IS POSSIBLY OUR FAVOURITE LUNCH RECIPE – IT'S A BEAUTY. YOU COULD ALWAYS SERVE IT WITHOUT THE GUACAMOLE, TO REDUCE YOUR FAT INTAKE, BUT WE LOVE IT TOO MUCH TO LEAVE IT OUT. BUT IT'S GOOD TO HAVE THE OPTION THOUGH.

SERVES 2

2 garlic cloves, crushed
2 teaspoons olive oil
1 teaspoon ground cumin
1 teaspoon smoked paprika
Juice of 1 lime
350g rump steak, fat trimmed
Sea salt and black pepper

FOR THE GUACAMOLE*

2 spring onions, finely chopped
1 green chilli, deseeded and
    finely chopped
1 small garlic clove, crushed
Juice of 1 lime
1 ripe medium avocado (150g)
Small bunch of coriander (25g),
    finely chopped
Sea salt and black pepper

TO SERVE

4 **small** soft flour tortillas
Chilli sauce

Preheat a griddle pan over a high heat. Combine the garlic, oil, spices and lime juice in a bowl then add the steak and toss to coat. Season the steak with salt and pepper then griddle for 2–3 minutes on each side. Transfer to a board to rest for 5 minutes.

Meanwhile make the guacamole. Combine the spring onions, chilli, garlic and lime juice in a bowl. Halve the avocado, scoop the flesh into the bowl and mash together with a fork. Stir in the chopped coriander and season to taste.

Warm the tortillas in a dry frying pan for 30 seconds until soft, then top each with some of the guacamole. Slice the steak thinly, pile on top of the guacamole and serve with chilli sauce.

PER SERVING: (*without guacamole)
KCAL: **243** (*168)   FAT: **12g** (*6g)
CARBS: **12g** (*7g)   PROTEIN: **21g** (*20g)

PER TORTILLA:
KCAL: **70**   FAT: **1.5g**
CARBS: **1.3g**   PROTEIN: **1g**

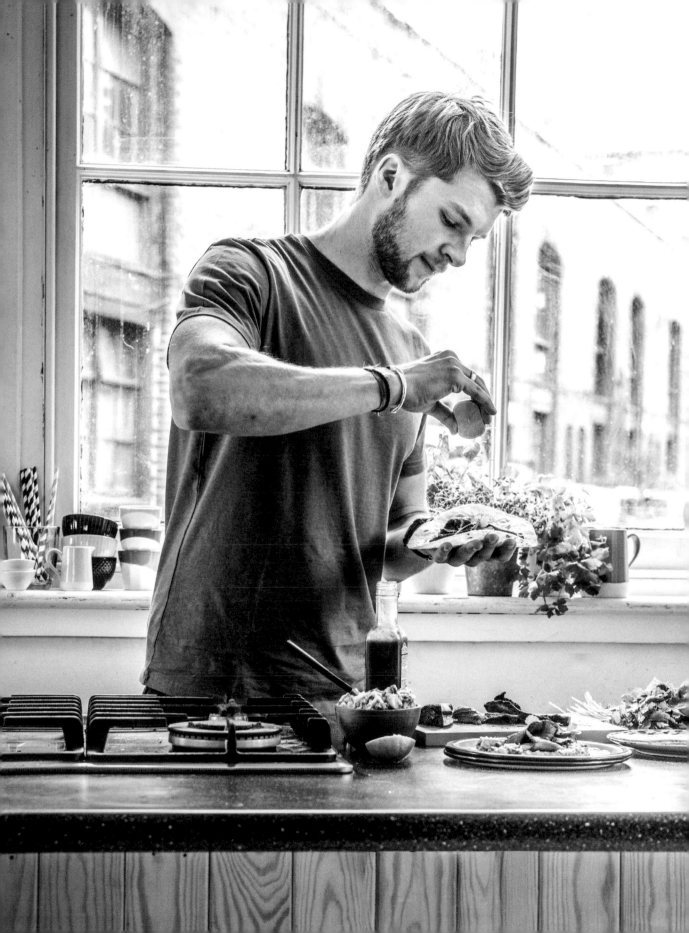

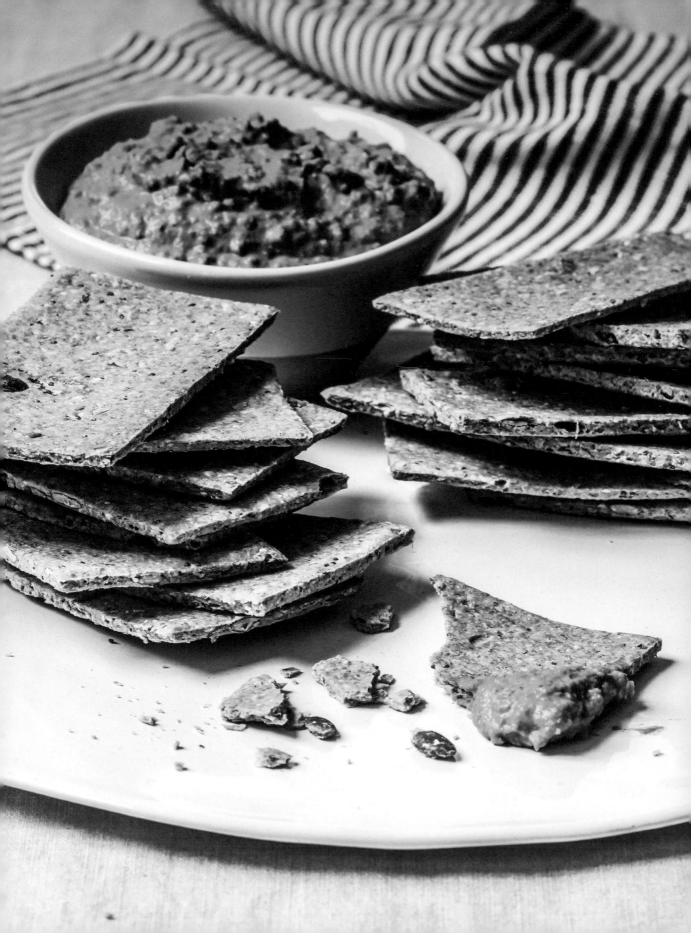

SEEDED SPELT CRACKERS

THIS HOMEMADE CRACKER RECIPE IS DELICIOUS AND INCREDIBLY VERSATILE – YOU CAN PRETTY MUCH SERVE THESE ALONGSIDE ANYTHING, OR JUST PACK UP A FEW IN AN AIRTIGHT CONTAINER FOR A LITTLE SNACK DURING THE DAY. VERSATILITY IS KEY WHEN YOU'RE EMBARKING ON A HEALTHY EATING JOURNEY. TRY SERVING THEM WITH OUR ROASTED RED PEPPER HOUMOUS ON PAGE 102.

MAKES 24

100g rolled oats
250g spelt flour
½ teaspoon baking powder
½ teaspoon fine sea salt
3 tablespoons flaxseed
3 tablespoons pumpkin seeds
2 tablespoons poppy seeds
4 tablespoons coconut oil, melted
135ml water

Preheat the oven to 150°C/gas mark 2.

Pour the oats into a food processor and blend to a coarse powder. Tip into a bowl and stir in the spelt flour, baking powder and salt.

Mix the seeds together in a separate bowl then add to the flour mix. Make a well in the middle of the flour mixture, pour in the coconut oil then gradually stir in the water until the mixture forms a stiff dough. Turn out onto a clean work surface and knead until you have a smooth ball.

Lay the dough between two sheets of baking parchment and roll out as thinly as possible into a rectangle roughly 40x30cm. Trim the edges to make a neat rectangle then, using a pizza cutter or sharp knife, cut the dough lengthways into six equal strips. Cut in half widthways, then in half again to make 24 rectangles.

Lay the sheet of crackers on a large baking tray and bake for 30 minutes until crisp. Leave to cool completely then store in an airtight container.

PER CRACKER:
KCAL: 88   FAT: 4g
CARBS: 10g   PROTEIN: 2g

ROASTED RED PEPPER HOUMOUS

EVERYONE LOVES A GOOD DIP WHEN FRIENDS ARE ROUND, AND THIS LITTLE SHOWSTOPPER IS ALWAYS GOOD TO HAVE IN YOUR ARMOURY. PEOPLE FORGET JUST HOW EASY DIPS ARE TO MAKE AND THERE ARE SO MANY COMBINATIONS TO SUIT YOU. YOU CAN SERVE THIS WITH EITHER STRIPS OF CARROT AND CUCUMBER OR SOME CRACKERS – TRY THE SEEDED SPELT CRACKERS ON PAGE 101.

SERVES 4 AS A SNACK

2 medium red peppers

1 red chilli

2 garlic cloves, unpeeled

1 x 400g tin chickpeas,
  rinsed and drained

2 tablespoons tahini

1 tablespoon olive oil

1 teaspoon ground cumin

1 teaspoon hot smoked paprika

Juice of 1 lemon

Sea salt and black pepper

Preheat the grill to its highest setting. Cut the peppers in half, remove the seeds and stalks and lay on a baking tray, cut side down. Add the chilli and garlic to the tray and grill for 15 minutes until the skins are blistered. Transfer the peppers to a bowl, cover with cling film and leave to stand for 10 minutes.

When the peppers are cool enough to handle peel them and put the flesh into a food processor. Peel the garlic and remove the stalk from the chilli and add to the food processor (you can deseed the chilli if you prefer your houmous to have less of a kick). Blend the peppers until smooth, then add the remaining ingredients and pulse to a rough paste. Season to taste and serve with crudités or toasted pitta bread for dipping.

PER SERVING:
KCAL: 185   FAT: 9g
CARBS: 20g   PROTEIN: 6g

SMOKED MACKEREL PÂTÉ

A GREAT ALL-ROUNDER, PARTICULARLY IF YOU WANT TO BOOST YOUR CALORIES, FAT AND PROTEIN CONTENT FOR THE DAY.

SERVES 2

2 smoked mackerel fillets (220g), skinned

100g full-fat cream cheese

2 tablespoons soured cream

2 teaspoons creamed horseradish (optional)*

Zest and juice of ½ lemon

Sea salt and black pepper

Flake two-thirds of the mackerel into a food processor, add the remaining ingredients and pulse until blended but not completely smooth.

Transfer to a bowl and flake in the remaining mackerel. Season to taste and serve with toast or Protein Flatbreads (see page 105).

PER SERVING: (*without horseradish)
KCAL: 570 (*530)   FAT: 48g (*45g)
CARBS: 5g (*4g)   PROTEIN: 29g (*28g)

BABA GANOUSH

A GREAT DIP TO HAVE WITH A MEAL OR AS A SNACK WITH SLICED PEPPERS, CARROT STICKS OR PITTA BREAD, FOR A SLIGHTLY HIGHER CARB OPTION. TRY THEM WITH OUR PROTEIN FLATBREADS AS WELL (SEE PAGE 105).

SERVES 4 AS A SNACK

2 large aubergines (800g)

1 garlic clove, crushed

2 tablespoons tahini

1 teaspoon smoked paprika

Juice of 1 lemon

Sea salt

Preheat the grill to its highest setting. Lay the aubergines on a baking tray and grill for 20 minutes, turning occasionally, until the skins are charred all over and the aubergines are starting to collapse. Set aside until cool enough to handle.

Cut the aubergines in half and scoop the flesh out with a spoon; make sure you get rid of any burnt bits. Put the aubergine flesh into a food processor with the remaining ingredients and pulse to a rough paste. Season to taste and serve with crudités or toasted pitta bread for dipping.

PER SERVING:
KCAL: 123   FAT: 6g
CARBS: 13g   PROTEIN: 4g

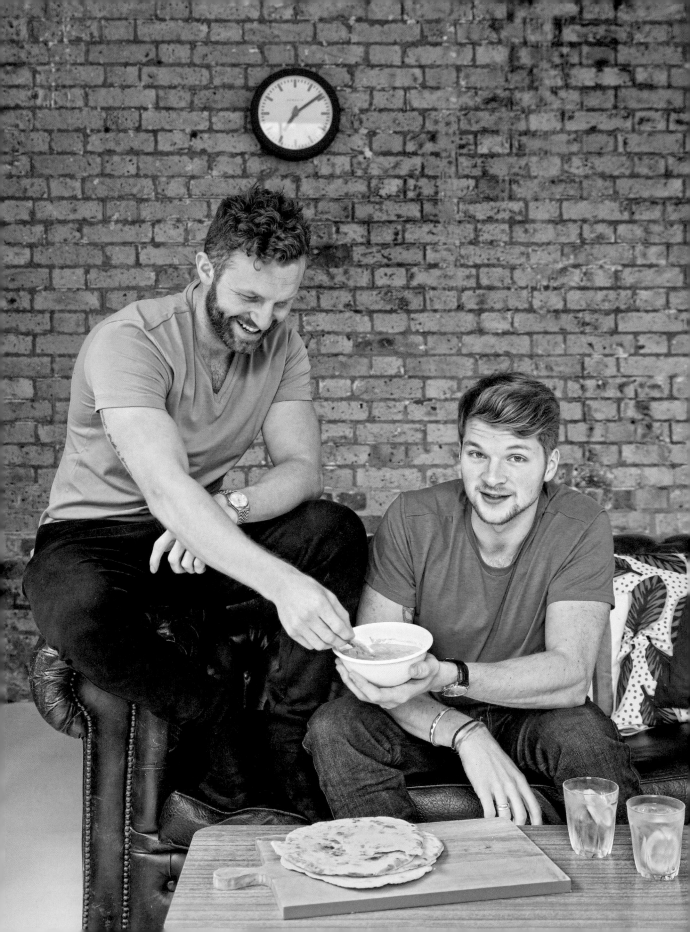

PEA, FETA + BASIL DIP

A GREAT DIP FOR WHEN YOU HAVE FRIENDS OR FAMILY ROUND AND YOU'RE STILL KEEPING AN EYE ON WHAT YOU'RE EATING.

SERVES 4 AS A SNACK

350g frozen peas

100g feta, crumbled

1 small garlic clove, crushed

Juice of ½ lemon

Small bunch of basil (20g)

Sea salt and black pepper

PER SERVING:
KCAL: 135   FAT: 5g
CARBS: 13g   PROTEIN: 9g

Bring a large pan of salted water to the boil, pour in the peas and cook for 3 minutes. Drain, reserving a little of the cooking water.

Tip the peas into a food processor and add the remaining ingredients. Blend until smooth, adding enough of the reserved cooking water to loosen to a smooth purée. Season to taste and then serve with crudités and the Seeded Spelt Crackers (see page 101).

PROTEIN FLATBREADS

THESE SIMPLE FLATBREADS, WITH ADDED PROTEIN POWDER, MAKE A GREAT SNACK, GIVING YOU A GOOD DOSE OF PROTEIN AS WELL AS CARBS. THEY ALSO FORM THE BASE OF OUR HAM AND MUSHROOM PIZZA (SEE PAGE 125). TRY THEM WITH ANY OF OUR DELICIOUS DIPS.

MAKES 4 BREADS

350g self-raising flour, plus extra
    for dusting

120g plain whey protein powder

1 teaspoon baking powder

½ teaspoon fine sea salt

300g natural yoghurt

PER BREAD:
KCAL: 234   FAT: 4g
CARBS: 32g   PROTEIN: 18g

Combine the flour, whey protein powder, baking powder and salt in a large bowl and make a well in the middle. Pour in the yoghurt and stir with a fork to combine. When the mixture forms a rough dough, turn out onto a lightly floured work surface and knead to form a smooth ball. Divide the dough into four equal pieces and roll each out into a thin circle around 10–15cm in diameter.

Heat a large frying pan over a high heat and cook the flatbreads one at a time for 2 minutes on each side until puffed up and starting to blister. As soon as each flatbread is ready, transfer it to a plate and cover with a clean tea towel to trap in the steam and soften the breads as they cool.

TRAIL MIX

THIS TRAIL MIX IS A GREAT LITTLE SNACK TO PACK UP AND SERVE OVER A FEW DAYS. JUST REMEMBER – AS WITH ALL NUT MIXES – IT IS VERY CALORIFIC, SO DON'T GET TOO CARRIED AWAY.

SERVES 8 AS A SNACK

75g unsalted cashew nuts

75g Brazil nuts, roughly chopped

75g blanched hazelnuts

75g coconut flakes

100g dried banana chips

100g dark chocolate chips

50g crystallised ginger, finely chopped

Preheat the oven to 180°C/gas mark 4.

Tip the nuts and coconut flakes onto a baking tray and spread out in an even layer. Bake for 10 minutes, shaking halfway through, until lightly toasted. Set aside to cool completely then tip into a large bowl. Add the remixing ingredients and stir to combine.

Transfer to a clip-top jar or airtight container and keep for up to a month.

PER SERVING:
KCAL: 397   FAT: 29g
CARBS: 28g   PROTEIN: 6g

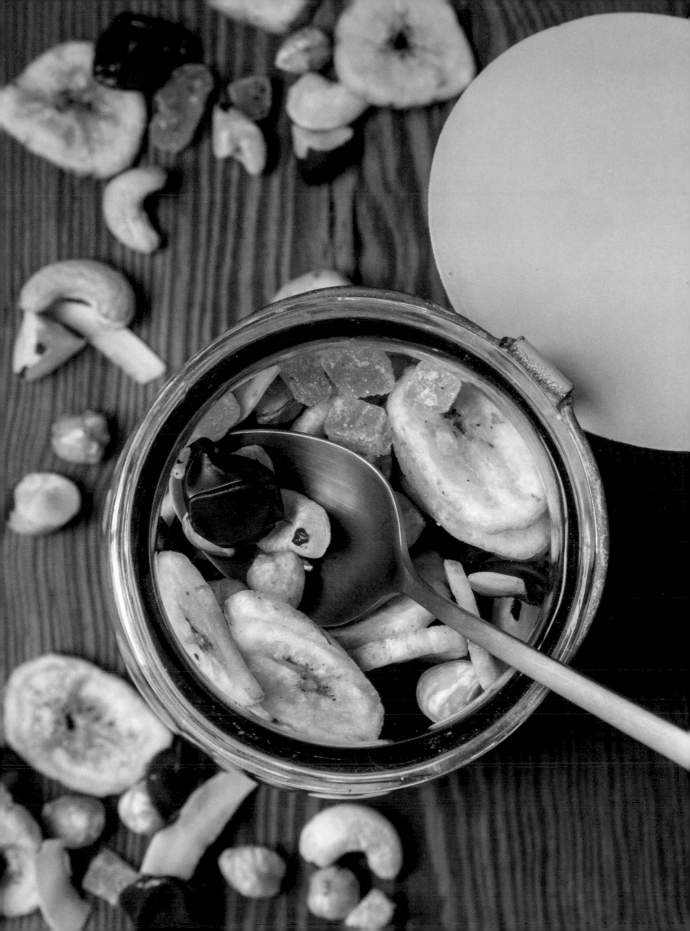

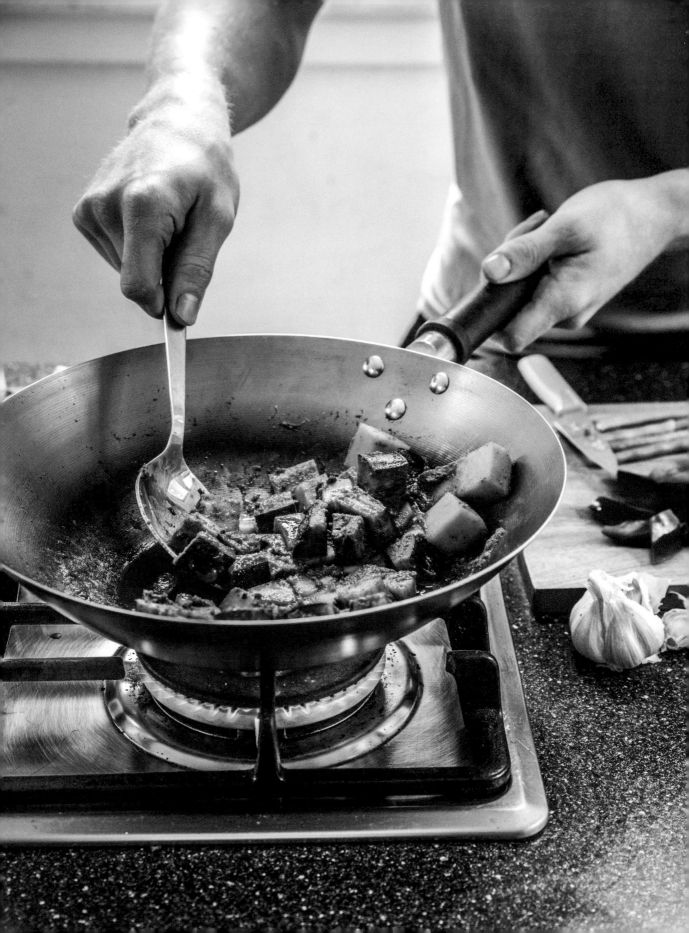

THAI RED VEGETABLE CURRY

WHILE WE WERE OFF TRAVELLING AROUND SOUTH EAST ASIA, WE BECAME BIG FANS OF THAI RED CURRY. THIS VERSION HAS GOT A LOVELY LITTLE KICK TO IT AND, WITH 350 CALORIES PER SERVING, IT'S AN ALL-ROUND WINNER IN OUR EYES. IF YOU'RE FEELING PARTICULARLY HUNGRY SERVE WITH 60G OF JASMINE RICE (DRIED WEIGHT) PER PERSON, WHICH WILL ADD AN EXTRA 212 CALORIES, 47G OF CARBS AND 4G OF PROTEIN PER SERVING TO HELP YOU FEEL FULLY SATISFIED.

SERVES 4

2 tablespoons coconut oil

2 tablespoons Thai red curry paste

500g small butternut squash, peeled, deseeded and cut into 2cm chunks

1 small aubergine, cut into 2cm chunks

1 x 400ml tin coconut milk

1 teaspoon palm sugar

1 medium red pepper, deseeded and cut into 2cm dice

120g green beans, trimmed and halved

1 x 225g tin bamboo shoots, drained

Juice of 1 lime

1 tablespoon fish sauce (or pinch of salt if you're vegetarian/vegan)

Small bunch of coriander (25g), leaves chopped

Heat the coconut oil in a wok or deep frying pan, add the curry paste and squash and fry for 3 minutes until fragrant. Add the aubergine and 200ml boiling water and cook for 5 minutes until the vegetables begin to soften.

Pour in the coconut milk and palm sugar, bring to the boil then cover and simmer gently for 10 minutes until the squash is tender. Add the red pepper, green beans and bamboo shoots, cook for a further 5 minutes then remove from the heat and stir in the lime juice, fish sauce (if using) and coriander. Serve as it is or with steamed rice.

PER SERVING:
KCAL: 350   FAT: 28g
CARBS: 22g   PROTEIN: 4g

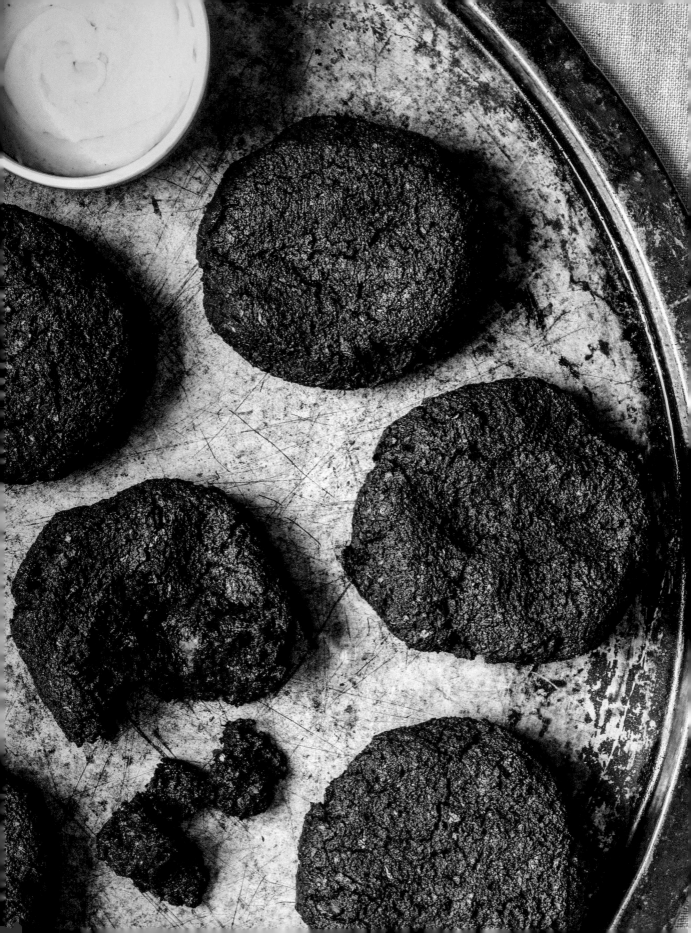

BEETROOT FALAFEL WITH TAHINI YOGHURT SAUCE

THIS IS A GREAT LOW-CALORIE MEAL, OR YOU COULD EVEN EAT THESE AS A HEALTHY SNACK, DEPENDING ON YOUR DAILY CALORIE GOALS.

SERVES 4

Olive oil spray

1 small red onion, chopped

2 garlic cloves, chopped

Small bunch of coriander (25g), roughly chopped

250g fresh beetroot, peeled and grated

1 x 400g tin chickpeas, rinsed and drained

3 tablespoons dry white breadcrumbs (20g)

1 teaspoon ground cumin

1 teaspoon smoked paprika

Sea salt and black pepper

FOR THE SAUCE

3 tablespoons Greek yoghurt

1 tablespoon tahini

2 teaspoons extra-virgin olive oil

Squeeze of lemon juice

TO SERVE

4 wholemeal pitta breads, toasted

2 baby gem lettuce, shredded

2 ripe tomatoes, thinly sliced

Preheat the oven to 160°C/gas mark 3, line a baking tray with baking parchment and lightly spray with olive oil.

Put the onion, garlic, coriander and beetroot into a food processor and blitz until smooth. Add the remaining ingredients and pulse to a coarse paste. Season to taste then shape into 12 small balls. Lay on the lined tray, spray lightly with olive oil and bake for 35 minutes. Meanwhile whisk together the ingredients for the sauce and season to taste.

Stuff the pitta breads with the falafel, lettuce and tomatoes and drizzle over the sauce.

PER SERVING:
KCAL: 387   FAT: 13g
CARBS: 52g   PROTEIN: 17g

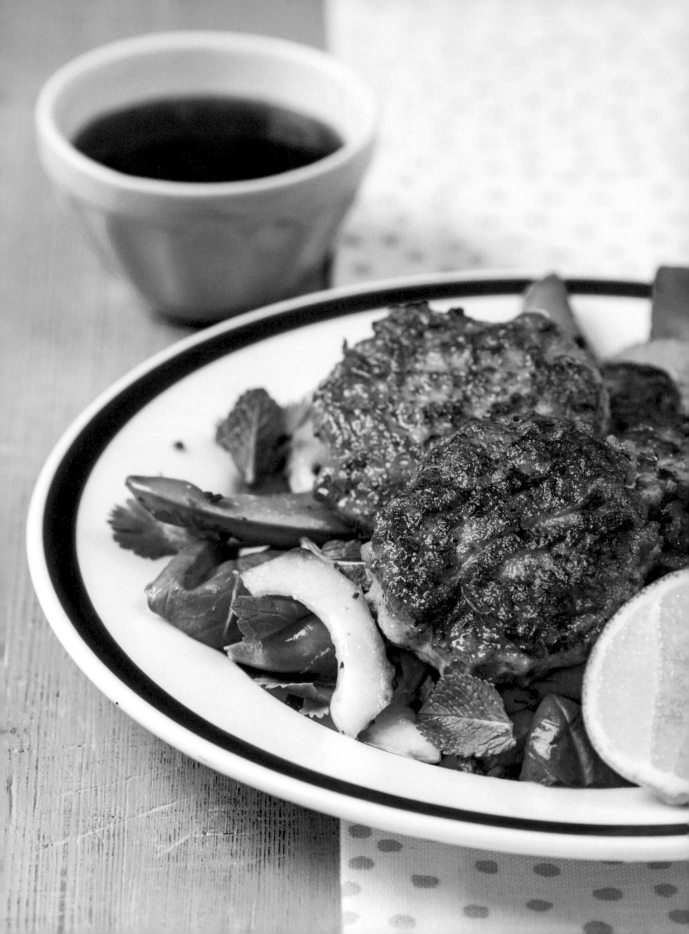

THAI FISH CAKES WITH CHILLI + HERB SALAD

SERVES 2

200g white fish fillet such as cod*, haddock or pollock, roughly chopped

100g (peeled weight) peeled and deveined raw tiger prawns, roughly chopped

2 tablespoons Thai red curry paste

Finely grated zest of 1 lime

50g green beans, finely chopped

½ small bunch of coriander (15g), finely chopped

2 tablespoons coconut oil

FOR THE SALAD

2 tablespoons rice vinegar

2 teaspoons palm sugar

1 garlic clove, finely chopped

1 Thai red chilli, finely chopped

½ cucumber, peeled, deseeded and sliced

200g sugar snap peas

Small bunch of mint (25g), leaves torn

Small bunch of coriander (25g), leaves torn

Small bunch of basil (25g), leaves torn

TO SERVE

2 tablespoons sweet chilli sauce

Juice of 1 lime

THESE THAI FISHCAKES SERVED WITH A HERBY SALAD MAKE SUCH A TASTY MEAL – DEFINITELY NOT YOUR REGULAR 'DIET' FOOD! THE CALORIES PER SERVING ARE PRETTY LOW BUT THE FLAVOUR LEVEL IS OFF THE CHART! IF FISHCAKES ARE NOT YOUR THING DO STILL TRY THE SALAD, WHICH COMES IN AT 140–160 CALORIES PER SERVING, AND ADD YOUR PREFERRED PROTEIN SOURCE.

Put the fish, prawns, curry paste and lime zest into a food processor and pulse until smooth and well combined. Tip into a bowl and stir in the beans and coriander. Using wet hands, shape the mixture into eight small fishcakes.

For the salad, whisk together the vinegar, palm sugar, garlic and chilli in a large bowl until the palm sugar has dissolved. Add the remaining ingredients and toss to combine.

Heat the coconut oil in a frying pan over a medium heat, add the fishcakes and fry for 2 minutes on each side. Meanwhile stir together the sweet chilli sauce and lime juice. Serve the fishcakes with the salad and dipping sauce.

PER SERVING: (*using cod)
KCAL: 250   FAT: 17g
CARBS: 4g   PROTEIN: 20g

LINGUINE WITH PRAWNS + CHILLI

WE LOVE FLAVOURING DISHES WITH LEMON AND CHILLI; THEY WORK SO WELL TOGETHER AND ADD A GREAT PUNCH OF ZINGY CITRUS AND CHILLI HEAT TO LOW-CALORIE DISHES. THIS IS ONE TO COOK FOR YOUR PARTNER – THEY WILL BE IMPRESSED BUT IT'S REALLY VERY SIMPLE TO MAKE!

SERVES 2

150g dried linguine

1 tablespoon olive oil

1 garlic clove, crushed

1 red chilli, finely chopped

250g cherry tomatoes, halved

200g (peeled weight) peeled and deveined large raw tiger prawns

Finely grated zest of ½ lemon

Sea salt and black pepper

Bring a large pan of salted water to the boil, add the linguine and cook for 8–10 minutes until al dente (or according to the packet instructions).

Meanwhile, heat the oil in a large frying pan over a medium heat, add the garlic and chilli and fry gently for 2 minutes. Increase the heat, add the cherry tomatoes and cook for 4–5 minutes until they start to break down.

Add the prawns and cook for 1–2 minutes until they start to turn pink. Add a small ladleful of the pasta cooking water to the pan, leave to cook for a couple of minutes then drain the pasta and add to the pan. Toss everything together then remove from the heat and stir through the lemon zest. Season to taste and serve.

PER SERVING:
KCAL: 450   FAT: 9g
CARBS: 59g   PROTEIN: 33g

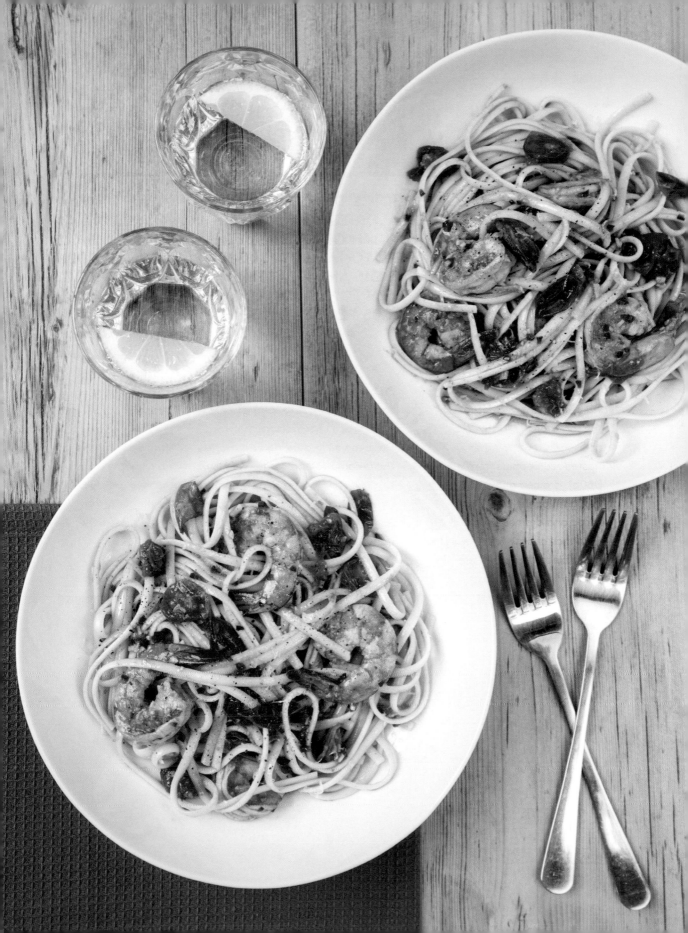

COD PARCELS WITH WHITE BEANS

A GREAT LOW-CALORIE CHOICE THAT DOESN'T SKIMP ON FLAVOUR. IF YOU WANT TO UP THE CALORIES WHY NOT ADD SOME SWEET POTATO WEDGES COOKED WITH OLIVE OIL AND PAPRIKA. ROUGHLY CHOP A MEDIUM SWEET POTATO (ABOUT 150G) INTO WEDGES, TOSS IN A TABLESPOON OF OLIVE OIL AND SCATTER WITH PAPRIKA. COOK IN A 200°C/GAS MARK 6 OVEN FOR 20–30 MINUTES. THIS WILL ADD 250 CALORIES AND 30G CARBS PER SERVING.

SERVES 2

1 tablespoon olive oil

1 small red onion, thinly sliced

1 garlic clove, crushed

3 ripe tomatoes (240g), diced

1 tablespoon tomato purée

2 roasted red peppers from a jar (160g), drained and sliced

1 x 400g tin cannellini beans, rinsed and drained

Small bunch of basil (25g), leaves torn

2 x 150g pieces thick-cut cod loin

Sea salt and black pepper

TO SERVE

Green salad (160g)

Preheat the oven to 200°C/gas mark 6 and cut two large square sheets (30x30cm) of baking parchment.

Heat the oil in a frying pan over a medium heat, add the onion and garlic and cook gently for 5 minutes until softened. Increase the heat, add the tomatoes and cook for 5 minutes until they start to break down. Stir in the tomato purée, peppers and beans and cook for a further 2–3 minutes. Stir in the basil and season to taste.

Spoon half of the bean mixture onto each piece of paper, just off centre and lay a piece of cod on top. Fold the paper over the top of the fish and fold the open edges over to make a neat parcel. Lay the parcels on a baking tray and cook in the oven for 15 minutes.

Unwrap the parcels and serve with a simple green salad.

PER SERVING:
KCAL: 300   FAT: 9g
CARBS: 20g   PROTEIN: 33g

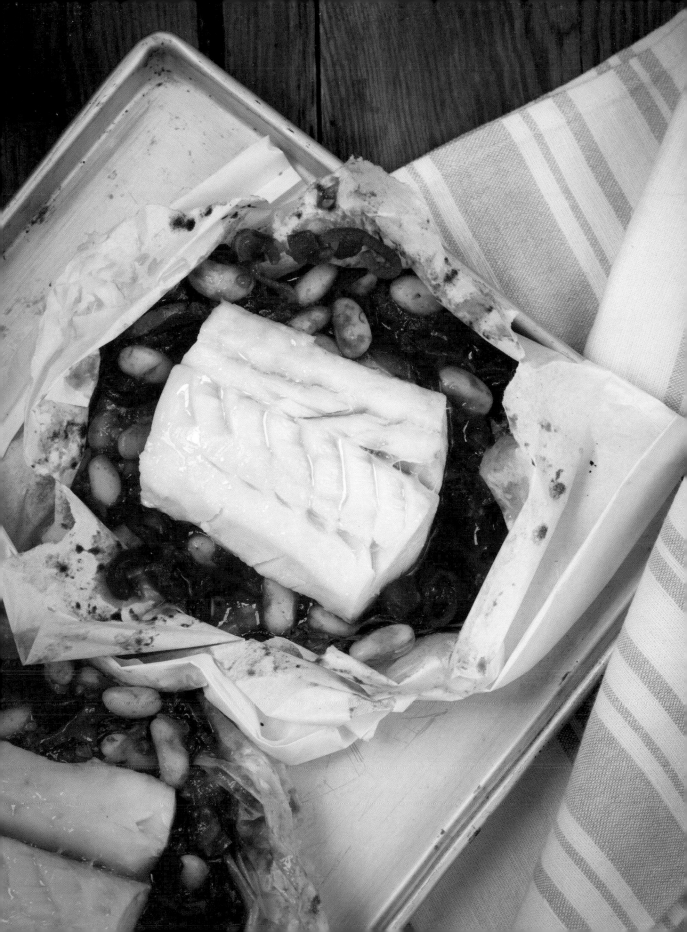

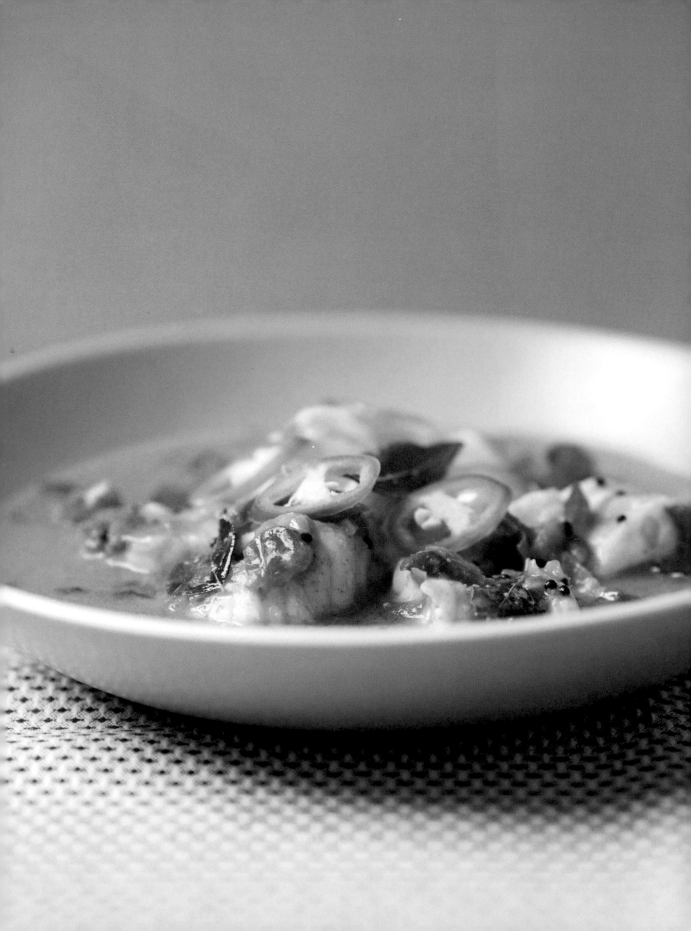

MONKFISH + COCONUT CURRY

CURRY IS ONE OF THOSE DISHES THAT MANY OF US ASSUME WE'LL NEVER BE ABLE TO CREATE AT HOME AS IT TAKES TOO MUCH EFFORT (AND OFTEN HAS ENDLESS INGREDIENTS). BUT THIS CURRY TASTES ABSOLUTELY DELICIOUS, IS EASY TO MAKE AND WILL BE A HIT WITH EVERYONE. DON'T BE PUT OFF BY THE CALORIES OR FAT CONTENT, WHICH ARE DOWN TO THE INCLUSION OF COCONUT MILK. IF YOU'RE A BIT WORRIED FEEL FREE TO USE LESS COCONUT MILK AND ADD A LITTLE WATER INSTEAD, OR USE REDUCED-FAT COCONUT MILK.

SERVES 2

1 tablespoon coconut oil

1 teaspoon black mustard seeds

1 tablespoon curry leaves

1 small onion, finely chopped

2 green chillies, sliced into thin rounds

2 garlic cloves, crushed

4cm piece of ginger, peeled and grated

1 teaspoon ground cumin

½ teaspoon ground turmeric

2 ripe tomatoes (120g), chopped

1 x 400ml tin coconut milk

200ml fish or vegetable stock

350g monkfish, cut into 3cm cubes

Sea salt

Heat the coconut oil in a deep frying pan, add the mustard seeds and curry leaves and fry gently for 2–3 minutes until the mustard seeds begin to pop. Add the onion and fry for 5 minutes until caramelised.

Add the chillies, garlic and ginger, fry for a minute then add the spices. Fry for a minute until fragrant then add the tomatoes and a splash of water. Fry for 3–4 minutes until the tomatoes begin to soften, then pour in the coconut milk and stock. Bring to a simmer then stir in the fish and cook gently for 5 minutes.

Season to taste and serve.

NOTES:

- For carb loading, serve with 125g cooked white or brown rice per person.
- For higher protein, add 150g peeled, raw tiger prawns at the same time as the monkfish.

PER SERVING:
KCAL: 605   FAT: 43g
CARBS: 20g   PROTEIN: 35g

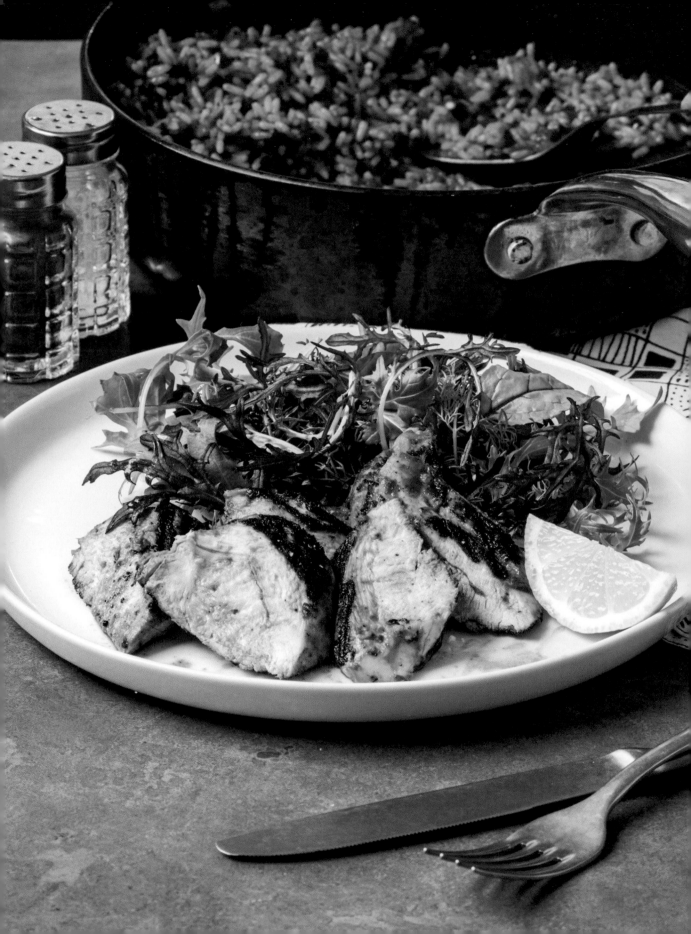

PIRI PIRI CHICKEN WITH SPICY RICE

ONE OF OUR FAVOURITE HOMEMADE MEALS, THIS TAKES MINIMAL TIME AND EFFORT TO COOK AND TASTES AMAZING. IF YOU FANCY A LOWER-CARB OPTION, SERVE WITHOUT THE SPICY RICE AND ADD 160G OF GREEN SALAD INSTEAD.

SERVES 2
2 x 170g skinless chicken breasts

FOR THE MARINADE
2 garlic cloves, crushed
3 red chillies, deseeded and
    finely chopped
Juice of ½ lemon
1 tablespoon red wine vinegar
2 teaspoons olive oil
2 teaspoons tomato purée (14g)
1 teaspoon dried oregano
1 teaspoon hot smoked paprika

FOR THE RICE
1 tablespoon olive oil
1 small onion, finely chopped
1 medium red pepper, deseeded
    and finely chopped
1 teaspoon ground cumin
1 x 250g pouch cooked long grain rice
Juice of ½ lemon
Sea salt and black pepper

TO SERVE
Lemon wedges

Lay the chicken breasts in a shallow dish and use a sharp knife to slash each breast a few times. Pour the marinade ingredients into a food processor, blend until smooth then pour over the chicken. Cover with cling film, put in the fridge and leave to marinate for at least half an hour, although overnight is best.

Remove the chicken from the fridge and pour any excess marinade into a small bowl. Heat the oil in a large frying pan over a medium heat, add the onion and pepper and fry for 10 minutes until softened. Add the reserved marinade and ground cumin, fry for a couple of minutes then add the rice and a splash of water. Fry for 3–4 minutes, then stir in the lemon juice and season to taste.

While the rice is cooking, heat a heavy-based griddle pan over a high heat. Lay the chicken in the pan and cook for 3–4 minutes on each side, or until cooked through.

Serve with the spicy rice (or a green salad) and the lemon wedges to squeeze over.

PER SERVING: (*with salad instead of rice)
KCAL: 543 (*250)   FAT: 20g (*10g)
CARBS: 46g (*3g)   PROTEIN: 42g (*38g)

MOROCCAN TURKEY KEBABS WITH CHICKPEA SALAD

KEBABS HAVE A SLIGHTLY BAD REP, THANKS TO THEM BEING THE FAST FOOD OF CHOICE AFTER A CRAZY, ALCOHOL-FUELLED NIGHT. NO NEED TO WORRY WITH THIS HEALTHY, HOMEMADE ALTERNATIVE, WHICH USES LOW-FAT TURKEY BREAST AND IS SERVED WITH A SPICED CHICKPEA SALAD.

SERVES 2

1 tablespoon olive oil

2 garlic cloves, crushed

2 teaspoons ras el hanout spice mix

2 teaspoons harissa paste or
   chilli sauce

Juice of ½ lemon

Pinch of salt

300g diced turkey breast

1 medium red pepper, deseeded and
   cut into 3cm chunks

FOR THE SALAD

1 tablespoon olive oil

Juice of 1 lemon

1 teaspoon ground cumin

½ teaspoon sweet smoked paprika

1 small red onion, finely sliced

1 x 400g tin chickpeas,
   rinsed and drained

Small bunch of parsley (25g),
   finely chopped

Sea salt and black pepper

TO SERVE

125ml Greek yoghurt

For the kebabs, whisk together the olive oil, garlic, ras el hanout, harissa (or chilli sauce), lemon juice and salt in a large bowl. Add the turkey and pepper, stir to combine then cover with cling film. Transfer to the fridge for at least half an hour to marinate.

Preheat the grill to its highest setting and thread the turkey and peppers onto skewers. Grill for 8–10 minutes, turning halfway through cooking.

While the kebabs are cooking, make the salad. Whisk together the oil, lemon juice and spices in a large bowl. Add the onions and chickpeas then roughly mash the chickpeas with the back of a fork. Add the parsley, stir to combine and season to taste.

Serve the kebabs with the chickpea salad and Greek yoghurt.

PER SERVING: (*without yoghurt)
KCAL: 630 (*553)   FAT: 23g (*20g)
CARBS: 30g (*28g)   PROTEIN: 60g (*54g)

TERIYAKI CHICKEN SKEWERS WITH NOODLES + PAK CHOI

THESE TERIYAKI SKEWERS LOOK AND TASTE DELICIOUS SO BEWARE: YOU WILL BE LICKING YOUR FINGERS LONG AFTER THEY'RE GONE. A GREAT OPTION WITH THESE IS TO MAKE AND COOK A DOUBLE PORTION OF THE TERIYAKI CHICKEN AND PUT HALF IN AN AIRTIGHT CONTAINER TO TAKE TO WORK – THEY MAKE A GREAT HIGH-PROTEIN NIBBLE.

SERVES 2

125ml teriyaki sauce

1 tablespoon runny honey

1 tablespoon dark soy sauce

20g fresh ginger, peeled and finely grated

2 x 170g skinless chicken breasts, cut into 2cm chunks

4 spring onions, cut into 2cm lengths

FOR THE NOODLES

125g dried medium egg noodles

2 pak choi, leaves separated

1 tablespoon dark soy sauce

1 teaspoon sesame oil

1 red chilli, deseeded and finely chopped

2 teaspoons sesame seeds

Preheat the grill to its highest setting and line a baking tray with tin foil. Combine the teriyaki sauce, honey, soy sauce and ginger in a bowl, add the chicken and spring onions and stir to coat. Thread the chicken and spring onions onto skewers and lay on the baking tray.

Pour the remaining marinade into a small pan, bring to the boil then turn down to a low heat.

Grill the skewers for 7–8 minutes, turning and brushing with the marinade a couple of times during cooking.

While the chicken is cooking, bring a large pan of salted water to the boil. Add the noodles, cook for 3 minutes, then add the pak choi and cook for a further 2 minutes. Drain the noodles and pak choi and tip into a large bowl. Add the soy sauce, sesame oil, chilli and sesame seeds and toss to combine. Serve the chicken skewers with the noodles and pak choi on the side.

PER SERVING:
KCAL: 612   FAT: 16g
CARBS: 65g   PROTEIN: 51g

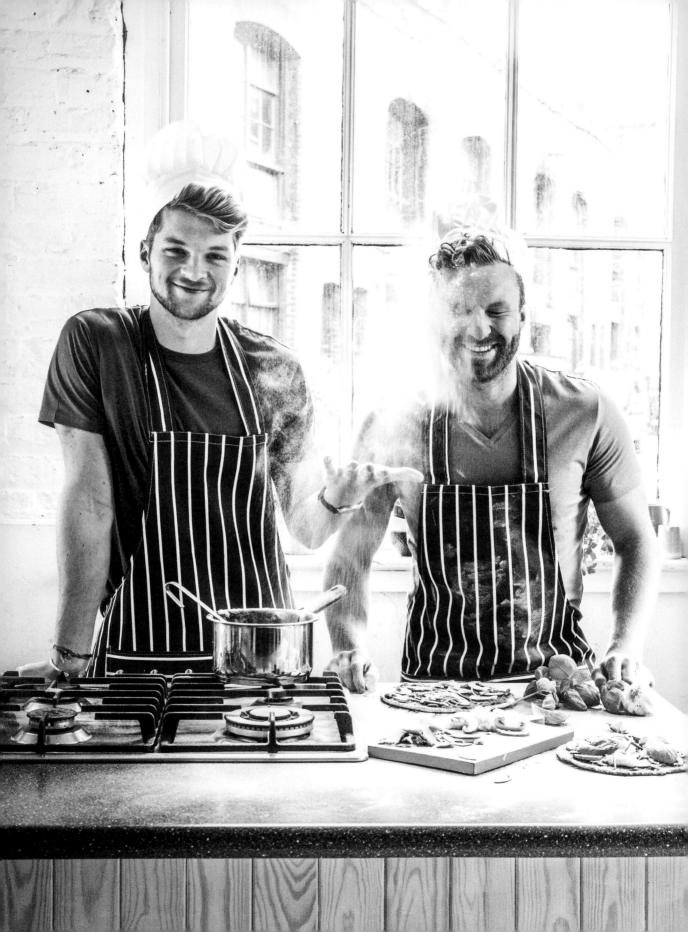

HAM + MUSHROOM PIZZA

THINK PIZZA BUT WITH MORE PROTEIN. THIS PIZZA IS IDEAL FOR THAT WELL-DESERVED MEAL AFTER A HARD WORKOUT, OR EVEN AS A SNACK IF CUT INTO SLICES.

SERVES 2

1 x 400g tin chopped tomatoes
1 teaspoon dried oregano
1 garlic clove, crushed
2 Protein Flatbreads (see page 105)
2 thick slices ham (40g),
   torn into chunks
4 chestnut mushrooms, thinly sliced
100g mozzarella,
   torn into small chunks
½ small red onion, thinly sliced
Sea salt and black pepper

Preheat the oven to its highest setting. While the oven is heating, pour the tinned tomatoes, oregano and garlic into a pan, bring to a simmer and cook gently for 10 minutes until thickened. Remove from the heat and season to taste.

Spread the sauce over the flatbreads then top with the ham, mushrooms, mozzarella and onion. Slide the pizzas onto two baking trays and bake for 10 minutes, or until the cheese is melted and bubbling. Leave to cool for a couple of minutes before serving.

PER PIZZA:
KCAL: <u>453</u>   FAT: <u>13g</u>
CARBS: <u>46g</u>   PROTEIN: <u>38g</u>

PAPRIKA PORK FILLET WITH BLACK LENTILS

THIS IS A GREAT HEARTY DINNER TO HAVE AT THE END OF A TRAINING DAY OR IN PREPARATION THE NIGHT BEFORE IF YOU ARE PLANNING TO FAST IN THE MORNING FOR A TRAINING SESSION – IT HAS A BIG KICK OF CARBS THAT WILL LOAD YOU UP. IF YOU WANT TO BRING THE CARBS DOWN, SIMPLY LEAVE OUT THE COOKED LENTILS – OR JUST HAVE A SMALLER PORTION.

SERVES 2

400g pork tenderloin fillet, sinew and excess fat trimmed (trimmed weight 300g)

2 teaspoons sweet smoked paprika

1 teaspoon fine sea salt

2 tablespoons olive oil

2 small red onions, thinly sliced

2 medium red peppers, deseeded and thinly sliced

2 garlic cloves, crushed

3 sprigs of thyme, leaves chopped

12 cherry tomatoes (150g), halved

1 x 250g pouch cooked black lentils

Small bunch of parsley (25g), roughly chopped

Preheat the oven to 200°C/gas mark 6.

Rub the pork all over with the paprika and salt. Heat 1 tablespoon of the oil in a large frying pan over a high heat, add the pork to the pan and sear for 2 minutes on each side; this is just to sear the outside of the meat, not to cook it through at this stage. Transfer the pork to a plate and set aside.

Heat the remaining oil in the pan then throw in the onions and peppers. Fry for 3 minutes then add the garlic, thyme and tomatoes and fry for a further 3 minutes.

Tip the vegetables into an ovenproof dish, lay the pork on top and cook in the oven for 15 minutes. Once the pork is cooked, remove the dish from the oven and lift the pork onto a warm plate to rest for 5 minutes. Meanwhile reheat the lentils according to the packet instructions then pour over the vegetables. Add the parsley and stir to combine.

Slice the rested pork and serve with the lentils.

PER SERVING:
KCAL: 539   FAT: 18g
CARBS: 40g   PROTEIN: 26g

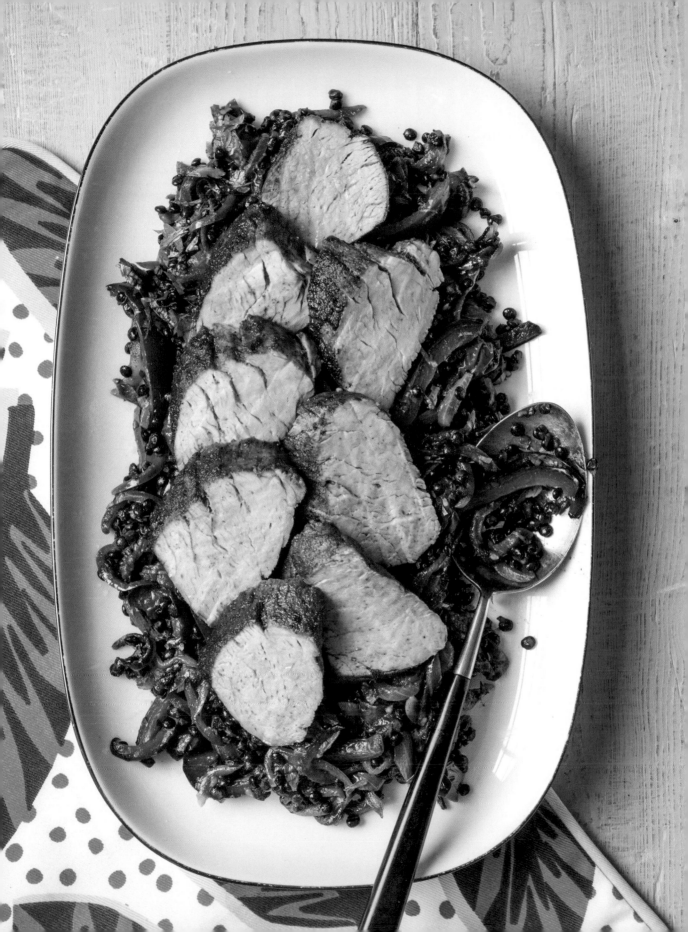

LAMB KEBABS WITH TZATZIKI

THERE'S A BIT OF GREEK INFLUENCE HERE WITH THE TZATZIKI, WHICH GOES SO WELL WITH THE LAMB. THIS IS SURE TO BECOME A FAVOURITE OF YOURS.

SERVES 2

1 tablespoon olive oil

1 garlic clove, crushed

1 teaspoon ground cumin

1 teaspoon dried oregano

1 teaspoon hot smoked paprika

350g diced lamb leg

1 medium red pepper, deseeded and diced

1 small red onion, cut into wedges

Sea salt and black pepper

FOR THE TZATZIKI

¼ cucumber, coarsely grated

½ garlic clove, crushed

1 teaspoon dried mint

125ml Greek yoghurt

TO SERVE

4 wholemeal pitta breads, toasted

2 ripe tomatoes, thinly sliced

Whisk together the oil, garlic, cumin, oregano and paprika in a large bowl, add the lamb, pepper and onion and toss to combine. Cover and chill for 1 hour or overnight if possible.

Remove the lamb from the fridge half an hour before cooking and season with salt and pepper. Preheat a griddle pan to a high heat. Thread the lamb onto skewers, alternating with pieces of pepper and onion. Griddle for 10 minutes, turning regularly, then set aside to rest for 5 minutes. Meanwhile combine the ingredients for the tzatziki in a bowl and season to taste.

Serve the lamb kebabs in warm pitta breads with the tzatziki and sliced tomatoes.

PER SERVING:
KCAL: 854   FAT: 46g
CARBS: 65g   PROTEIN: 45g

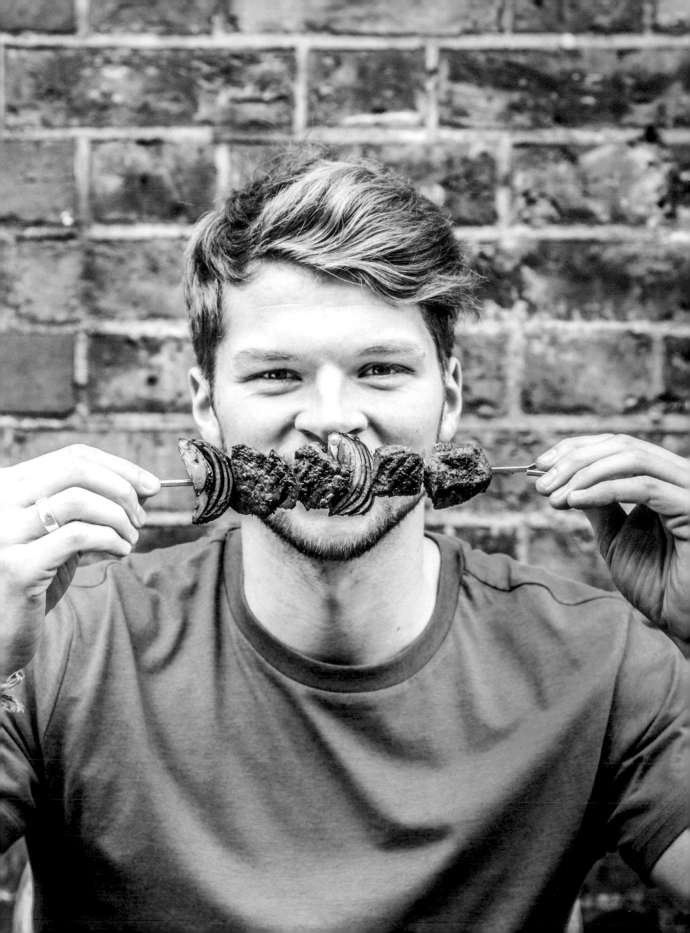

SHEPHERD'S PIE

THIS SHEPHERD'S PIE IS A REAL SHOWSTOPPER TO BRING OUT FOR FAMILY OR FRIENDS. IT PACKS A NICE CALORIE PUNCH SO YOU SURE WON'T BE LEFT WANTING DESSERT AFTERWARDS EITHER. THE SWEET POTATO TOPPING MAKES A GREAT CHANGE FROM REGULAR WHITE POTATOES.

SERVES 4

1 tablespoon coconut oil
2 small onions, finely chopped
2 carrots (200g), peeled and
  finely chopped
1 garlic clove, crushed
500g lean (10% fat) lamb mince
1 tablespoon tomato purée
4 sprigs of thyme, leaves chopped
400ml lamb or chicken stock
1 teaspoon Worcestershire sauce
1kg sweet potatoes, peeled
  and diced
25g butter
1 leek, finely sliced
Sea salt and black pepper

Heat the coconut oil in a heavy-based pan, add the onions, carrots and garlic and cook gently for 10 minutes until softened and caramelised. Increase the heat, add the lamb mince and fry for 5 minutes until golden.

Stir in the tomato purée and thyme, fry for a further 2 minutes then pour over the stock and Worcestershire sauce. Simmer gently, uncovered, for 30 minutes, stirring occasionally, until most of the liquid has evaporated. Season to taste and pour into a deep ovenproof dish, roughly 25x20cm.

Meanwhile preheat the oven to 180°C/gas mark 4 and bring a large pan of salted water to the boil. Add the sweet potatoes to the pan and cook for 10–12 minutes until soft. Drain thoroughly, then mash until smooth. Fry the leek in the butter for 5 minutes over a low-medium heat until soft, then stir into the sweet potato mash and season to taste.

Spoon the mash over the top of the lamb in an even layer then rough up the top with a fork. Cook in the oven for 30 minutes until the top of the mash is golden brown.

PER SERVING:
KCAL: 516   FAT: 16g
CARBS: 62g   PROTEIN: 31g

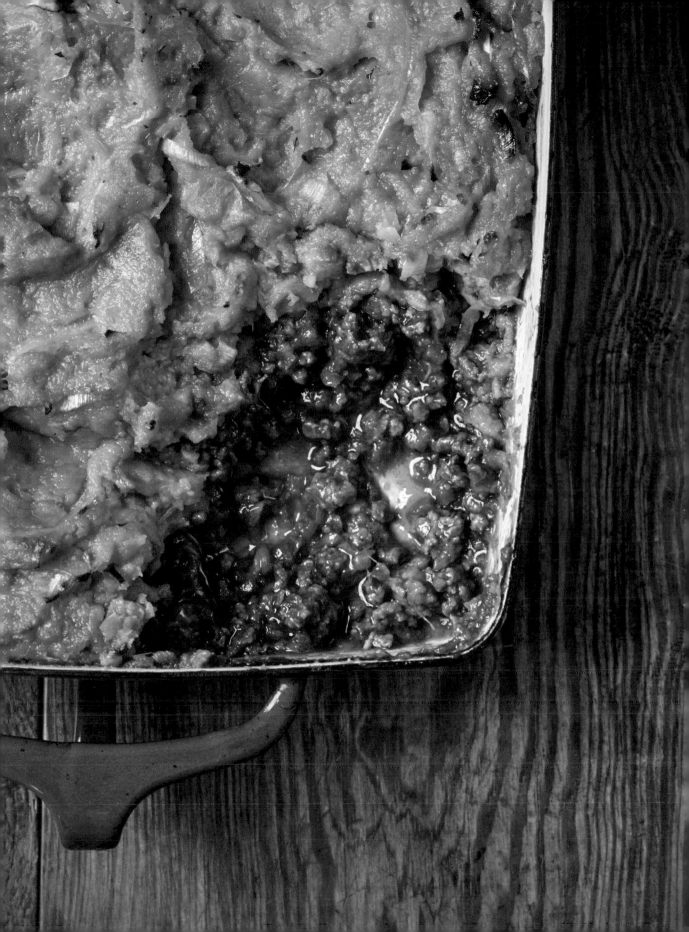

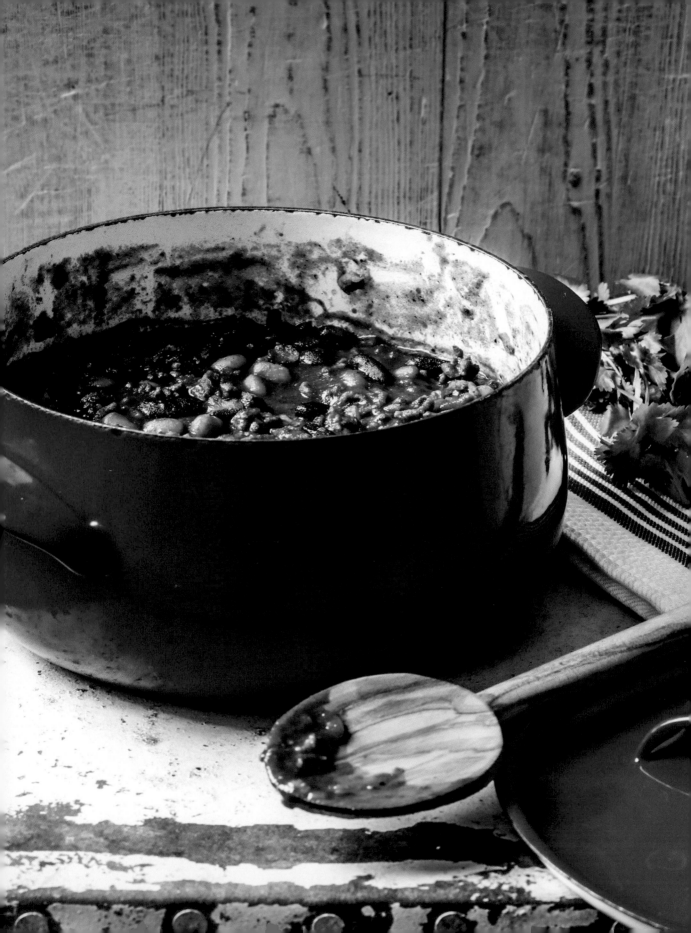

SLOW-COOKED BEEF CHILLI

WE ARE BIG FANS OF A GOOD, HEARTY CHILLI AND THIS IS SUPER SIMPLE, ESPECIALLY IF YOU OWN A SLOW COOKER – WE OFTEN DO THIS OVERNIGHT ON A SUNDAY AND THEN PORTION INTO PLASTIC CONTAINERS FOR THE WEEK AHEAD. ALTERNATIVELY, FREEZE INDIVIDUAL PORTIONS IN ZIPLOC FREEZER BAGS; STACK THEM ON TOP OF EACH OTHER AND THEN JUST TAKE OUT AND USE AS AND WHEN NEEDED. SIMPLY DEFROST THOROUGHLY AND REHEAT UNTIL PIPING HOT ALL THE WAY THROUGH.

SERVES 4

2 tablespoons olive oil

500g lean (5% fat) beef mince

1 large onion, finely chopped

1 garlic clove, crushed

1 teaspoon hot chilli powder

1 teaspoon ground cumin

½ teaspoon ground cinnamon

2 tablespoons tomato purée

500ml fresh beef stock

1 x 400g tin chopped tomatoes

1 x 400g tin kidney beans, rinsed and drained

1 x 400g tin baked beans

Sea salt and black pepper

Small bunch of coriander (25g), roughly chopped

Lime wedges to serve

Heat 1 tablespoon of the oil in a heavy-based pan or casserole dish, add the beef and fry for 5 minutes until browned. Remove the beef from the pan with a slotted spoon, transfer to a bowl and set aside.

Add the remaining oil to the pan then add the onion and fry for 5 minutes until softened. Add the garlic and spices, fry for 1 minute then add the tomato purée and fry for a further minute. Return the beef and any resting juices to the pan, add the stock and tomatoes and stir to combine. Cover and simmer gently for 45 minutes, stirring occasionally. Add the kidney beans and baked beans, cover and cook for a further 10 minutes; season to taste.

Top with the chopped coriander and serve with lime wedges.

NOTES:

- For a higher carb option, serve with either steamed rice or Flatbreads (see page 105), lightly grilled until crisp.

- For higher-fat version, add 150g chopped chorizo when you fry the onions and serve with 1 tablespoon soured cream or Greek yoghurt per serving.

PER SERVING:
KCAL: 425   FAT: 14g
CARBS: 22g   PROTEIN: 35g

CHILLI BEEF AVOCADO BURGERS

THESE ARE AMAZING! THEY ARE A GREAT LOW-CARB OPTION TO HAVE WITH GREEN VEG. MAKE SURE YOU USE LEAN (5% FAT) BEEF MINCE TO AVOID USING UP TOO MANY OF YOUR DAILY CALORIES – YOU ARE ALREADY GETTING PLENTY OF PROTEIN AND HEALTHY FATS FROM THE AVOCADO. THE LEMON JUICE AND CHILLI REALLY MAKE THESE SPECIAL SO DON'T BE TEMPTED TO LEAVE THEM OUT.

SERVES 2

400g lean (5% fat) beef mince

2 red chillies, deseeded and
    finely chopped

Sea salt and black pepper

1 ripe medium avocado (150g)

2 sundried tomatoes, finely chopped

Juice of 1 lemon

Combine the beef and half of the chopped chillies in a bowl, season with salt and pepper then divide into four balls. Flatten each into a thin patty and set aside.

Halve the avocados, scoop the flesh into a bowl and mash with a fork. Stir in the remaining chilli, the sundried tomatoes and the lemon juice. Put a tablespoon of the avocado mixture in the centre of two of the patties, then top each with the remaining patties. Press down the edges to seal the avocado in the middle of the burger.

Heat a griddle pan to a high heat, add the burgers and cook for 5 minutes on each side until cooked though.

PER SERVING:
KCAL: 404   FAT: 20g
CARBS: 13g   PROTEIN: 43g

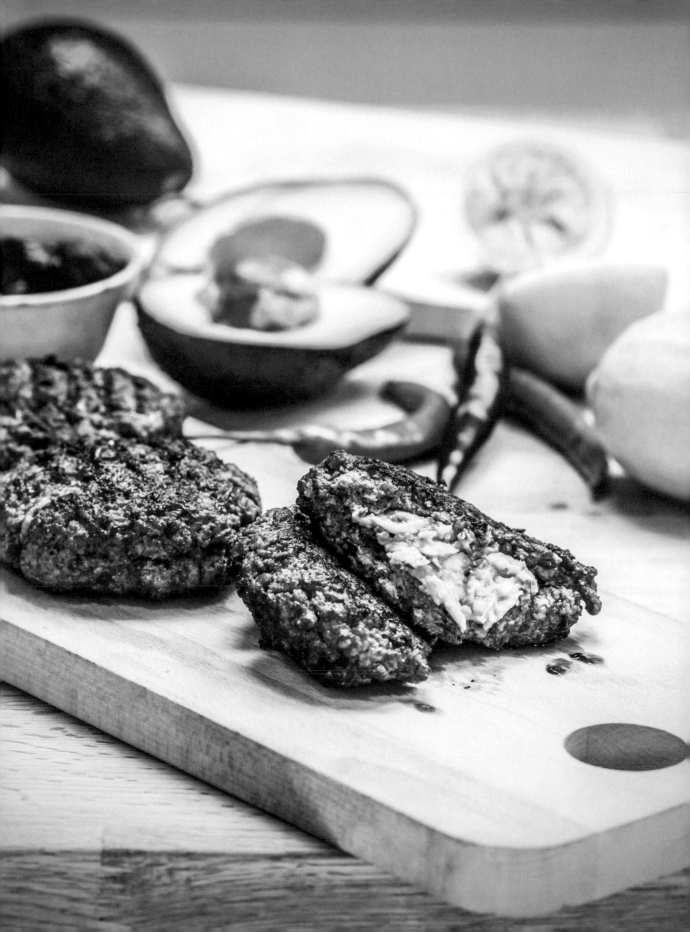

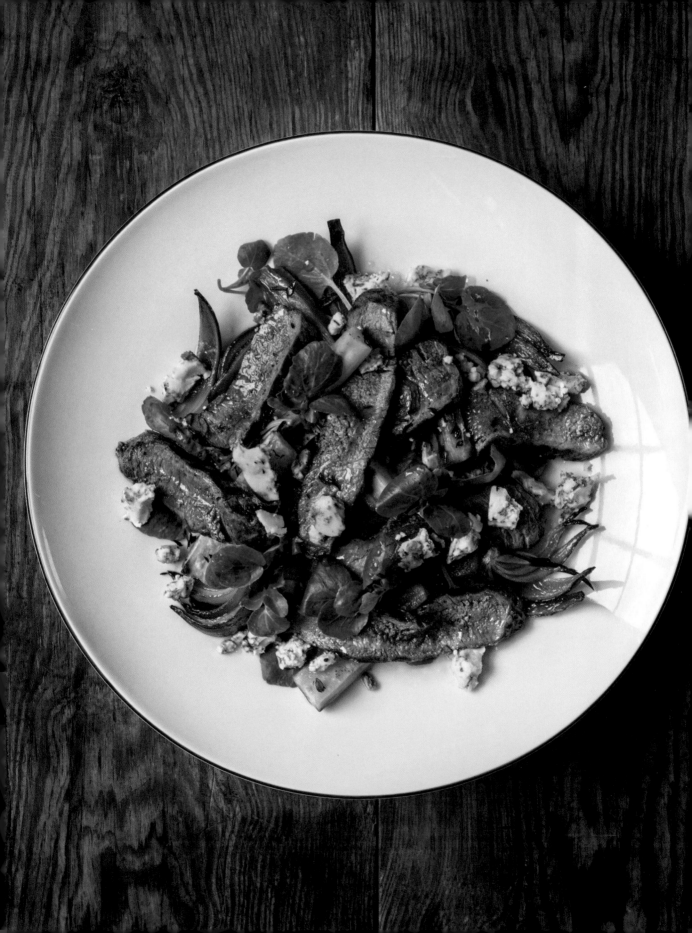

STEAK, ROAST VEGETABLE + BLUE CHEESE SALAD

WE LOVE A GOOD STEAK; HERE THE BLUE CHEESE SALAD ADDS A NEW DIMENSION TO THE CLASSIC STEAK WITH VEG. IF YOU'RE NOT A HUGE FAN OF BLUE CHEESE FEEL FREE TO USE A DIFFERENT CHEESE, OR, IF YOU'RE WATCHING YOUR CALORIE INTAKE, LEAVE THE CHEESE OUT ALL TOGETHER TO SAVE A GOOD 150–170 CALORIES PER SERVING. A GOOD LITTLE TIP IS TO PREPARE DOUBLE THE AMOUNT OF ROASTED VEGETABLES TO HAVE THE FOLLOWING DAY.

SERVES 2

2 parsnips (300g), peeled and cut into batons

2 small carrots (180g), peeled and cut into batons

1 small red onion, cut into wedges

3 garlic cloves, unpeeled and bashed

2 sprigs of thyme

1 tablespoon olive oil

Sea salt and black pepper

2 x 170–200g sirloin steaks, fat trimmed

Large bunch of watercress

2 teaspoons red wine vinegar

100g blue cheese (Stilton or Roquefort), crumbled

Preheat the oven to 200°C/gas mark 6.

Tip the parsnips, carrots, onion, garlic and thyme into roasting tin, drizzle over the oil and season with salt and pepper. Toss to combine then roast in the oven for 30 minutes, shaking occasionally during cooking.

When the vegetables are almost ready, preheat a griddle pan over a high heat. Season the steaks and griddle for 2–3 minutes on each side, or until cooked to your liking. Set aside to rest for 5 minutes.

Tip the vegetables into a large bowl and squeeze the garlic cloves out of their skins. Add the watercress, vinegar and cheese and gently toss to combine. Pile the salad onto a serving plate, cut the steak into slices and sit on top of the salad.

PER SERVING:

KCAL: 546   FAT: 30g
CARBS: 38g   PROTEIN: 31g

BEEF STIR FRY WITH RICE NOODLES

STIR-FRIES ARE A GREAT WAY TO GET LOADS OF COLOURFUL VEG INTO YOUR DIET, INCLUDING ONE OF OUR FAVOURITES: PEPPERS, WHICH ARE HIGH IN ANTIOXIDANTS. THIS RECIPE IS VERY WELL BALANCED WITH PLENTY OF PROTEIN, HOWEVER, YOU COULD REDUCE THE CARBS AND CALORIES BY SWAPPING THE NOODLES FOR A GREEN VEGETABLE, SUCH AS TENDERSTEM BROCCOLI.

SERVES 2

2 tablespoons coconut oil

400g lean beef stir-fry strips

2 garlic cloves, sliced

1 red chilli, deseeded and finely sliced

1 medium red pepper, deseeded and finely sliced

1 medium yellow pepper, deseeded and finely sliced

1 medium green pepper, deseeded and finely sliced

12 baby button mushrooms, sliced

200g cooked rice vermicelli noodles

2 tablespoons dark soy sauce

1 tablespoon rice vinegar

Heat a wok or large frying pan over a high heat until smoking, add half of the oil then brown half of the beef for a couple of minutes. Use a slotted spoon to transfer to a plate then repeat with the remaining oil and beef.

Add the garlic and chilli to the pan, fry for a minute then add the peppers. Fry over a high heat for 3 minutes, then add the mushrooms and a splash of water. Fry for a couple more minutes until the mushrooms have softened then return the beef to the pan along with any resting juices. Stir in the noodles, soy sauce and vinegar, cook for a further minute then divide between two bowls and serve.

PER SERVING:
KCAL: 510   FAT: 20g
CARBS: 44g   PROTEIN: 38g

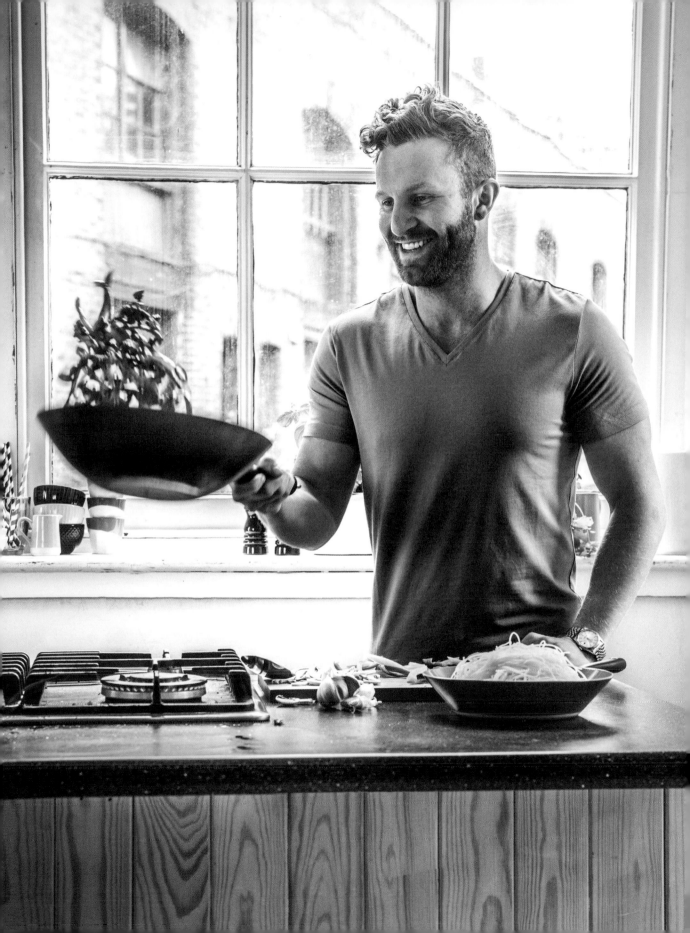

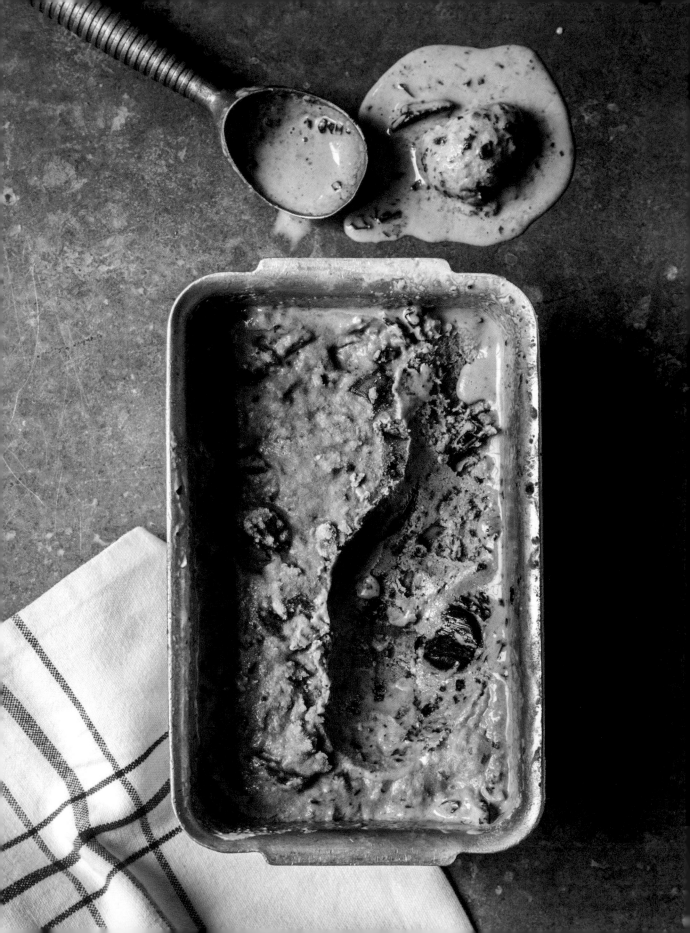

CHERRY CHOC CHIP FROZEN YOGHURT

IF YOU LOVE YOGHURT THEN THIS WILL BE RIGHT UP YOUR STREET: IT'S SWEET, EASY TO MAKE AND SIMPLE TO SEPARATE INTO PORTION SIZES TO SHARE OUT WITH FAMILY AND FRIENDS, OR JUST TO HAVE YOURSELF OVER THE COMING DAYS. IF YOU WANT A LITTLE EXTRA PROTEIN FEEL FREE TO ADD IN A SCOOP OF YOUR FAVOURITE PROTEIN POWDER (WITH AN AVERAGE OF 12–15G OF PROTEIN PER SCOOP IT WILL ADD AN EXTRA 10 CALORIES PER SERVING).

MAKES ABOUT 800ML

500g natural yoghurt

350g frozen pitted cherries

1 tablespoon runny honey

Juice of ½ lemon

100g dark chocolate (70% cocoa solids), finely chopped

Pour the yoghurt into a food processor with most of the cherries (reserve a handful for the end), the honey and lemon juice. Blend until smooth, then stir in the reserved cherries and the chopped chocolate.

Pour into a shallow plastic container and freeze for 30 minutes. Stir the mixture with a fork to break up any ice crystals then return to the freezer. Continue this process every 30 minutes until the mixture is smooth and set (it'll take between 3–4 hours in total). Serve on its own or topped with a handful of Granola (see page 63).

NOTE:

- We've used frozen cherries as they're cheaper and already pitted, plus it speeds up the freezing time.

PER SERVING: (based on 8 servings)
KCAL: 144   FAT: 8g
CARBS: 14g   PROTEIN: 4g

SWEET POTATO BROWNIES

WITH FEWER CALORIES THAN YOUR TYPICAL BROWNIE, THESE ARE A TREAT YOU CAN AFFORD TO INDULGE IN, THANKS TO THE PURÉED SWEET POTATO, WHICH ADDS SWEETNESS AND TEXTURE. THEY MAKE A LOVELY LITTLE SNACK OR DESSERT TO HAVE AFTER TEA ONE NIGHT. TRY THEM OUT – YOUR FRIENDS AND FAMILY WILL LOVE YOU FOREVER.

MAKES 12

1 ripe medium avocado (150g)

200g puréed sweet potato

125g apple sauce

75g runny honey

2 large free-range eggs

1 teaspoon vanilla extract

65g spelt flour

65g cocoa powder

60g chocolate whey protein powder

1 teaspoon baking powder

½ teaspoon fine sea salt

75g chopped walnuts

Preheat the oven to 190°C/gas mark 5 and line the base and sides of a 20cm square tin with baking parchment.

Cut the avocado in half and scoop the flesh into a food processor. Add the sweet potato, apple sauce, honey, eggs and vanilla extract and blend until smooth.

Sift the flour, cocoa powder, protein powder, baking powder and salt into a large bowl then stir in the wet mixture. Fold in the walnuts then spoon the mixture into the prepared tin. Bake for 25 minutes then transfer to a wire rack to cool in the tin. Turn out, cut into 12 rectangles and serve.

PER BROWNIE:
KCAL: 183   FAT: 8g
CARBS: 20g   PROTEIN: 8g

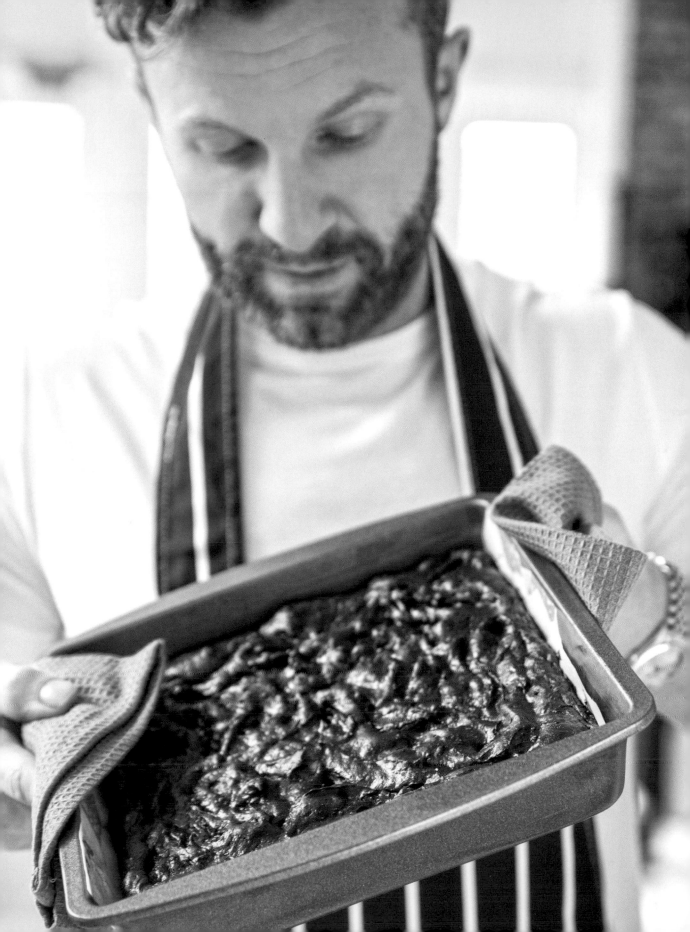

CHOCOLATE + ALMOND BUTTER MOUSSE

CHOCOLATE AND NUT BUTTER TOGETHER, WHAT MORE COULD YOU WANT? OKAY, A CHOCOLATE AND ALMOND BUTTER MOUSSE – BOOM!

SERVES 2

75g dark chocolate (70% cocoa solids)
1 tablespoon smooth almond butter
1 large free-range egg yolk
3 large free-range egg whites

Break the chocolate into small pieces and put into a heatproof bowl. Microwave on medium power for 30 seconds then stir. Continue to heat in 30-second bursts (it'll take 2–3 bursts, depending on how powerful your microwave is) until the chocolate has just melted; be careful not to overheat as the chocolate can burn easily. (Alternatively, if you don't have a microwave, you can set the bowl of chocolate over a pan of gently simmering water and stir until liquid.) While the chocolate is still warm, beat in the almond butter and egg yolk until smooth.

In a separate, clean bowl, whisk the egg whites to soft peaks. Whisk one-third of the egg whites into the chocolate mixture until smooth, then carefully fold in the remaining egg whites, keeping as much air in the mixture as possible.

Spoon the mixture into serving glasses or small bowls then chill for 2 hours until set.

PER SERVING:
KCAL: 296   FAT: 18g
CARBS: 23g   PROTEIN: 12g

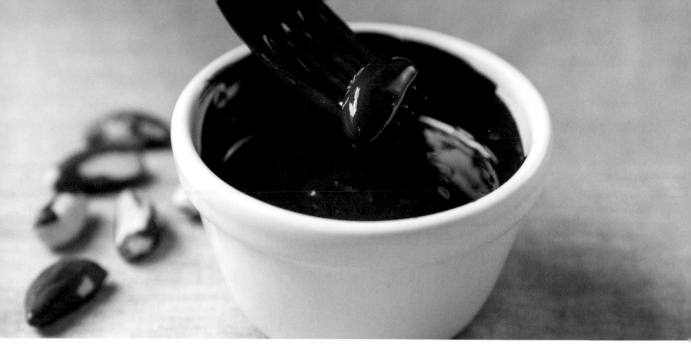

CHOCOLATE COATED NUTS

NAUGHTY NAUGHTY! WE ALL LIKE A TREAT EVERY NOW AND THEN AND WHAT COULD BE BETTER THAN THESE CHOCOLATE-COVERED NUTS. KEEP THE SERVING SIZE TO A SMALL HANDFUL TO AVOID WIPING OUT THE MAJORITY OF YOUR DAILY CALORIE ALLOWANCE IN ONE GO.

SERVES 8 AS A SNACK

100g dark chocolate (70% cocoa solids)
100g macadamia nuts
100g brazil nuts

Break the chocolate into small pieces and put into a heatproof bowl. Microwave on medium power for 30 seconds then stir. Continue to heat in 30-second bursts (it'll take 2–3 bursts, depending on how powerful your microwave is) until the chocolate has just melted; be careful not to overheat as the chocolate can burn easily. (Alternatively, if you don't have a microwave, you can set the bowl of chocolate over a pan of gently simmering water and stir until liquid.) Add the nuts and stir until evenly coated.

Line a baking tray with baking parchment then use a fork to remove the nuts from the chocolate and let any excess drip off. Lay the nuts on the lined tray, keeping them spaced apart so that they don't stick together as they set. Set aside to cool and set at room temperature for half an hour then chill in the fridge until firm.

PER SERVING:
KCAL: 247 **FAT:** 23g
CARBS: 9g **PROTEIN:** 4g

PROTEIN BALLS

THE BELOVED PROTEIN BALL. WE'VE SEEN SO MANY VARIATIONS OF THESE CHEEKY LITTLE NUMBERS OVER THE YEARS SO HERE IS OUR VERSION. IT'S A GREAT LITTLE CALORIE KICK AND PICK-ME-UP, TO HELP YOU AVOID THE TRIP TO THE SHOP TO GRAB AN ENERGY DRINK OR CHOCOLATE BAR. THEY TASTE AMAZING TOO!

MAKES 12

75g dark chocolate (70% cocoa solids)
125g almond butter
100g rolled oats
100g runny honey
75g chopped mixed nuts
2 tablespoons desiccated coconut
2 tablespoons flaxseed
1 scoop plain or vanilla whey protein powder (30g)

Break the chocolate into small pieces and put into a heatproof bowl. Microwave on medium power for 30 seconds then stir. Continue to heat in 30-second bursts (it'll take 2–3 bursts, depending on how powerful your microwave is) until the chocolate has just melted; be careful not to overheat as the chocolate can burn easily. (Alternatively, if you don't have a microwave, you can set the bowl of chocolate over a pan of gently simmering water and stir until liquid.)

Combine the melted chocolate with all of the remaining ingredients in a food processor and pulse to a coarse paste. Using slightly wet hands, roll the mixture into 12 equal-sized balls and transfer to a plate or baking tray. Wrap individually in cling film and chill for 2 hours.

PER BALL:
KCAL: 243   FAT: 15g
CARBS: 20g   PROTEIN: 7g

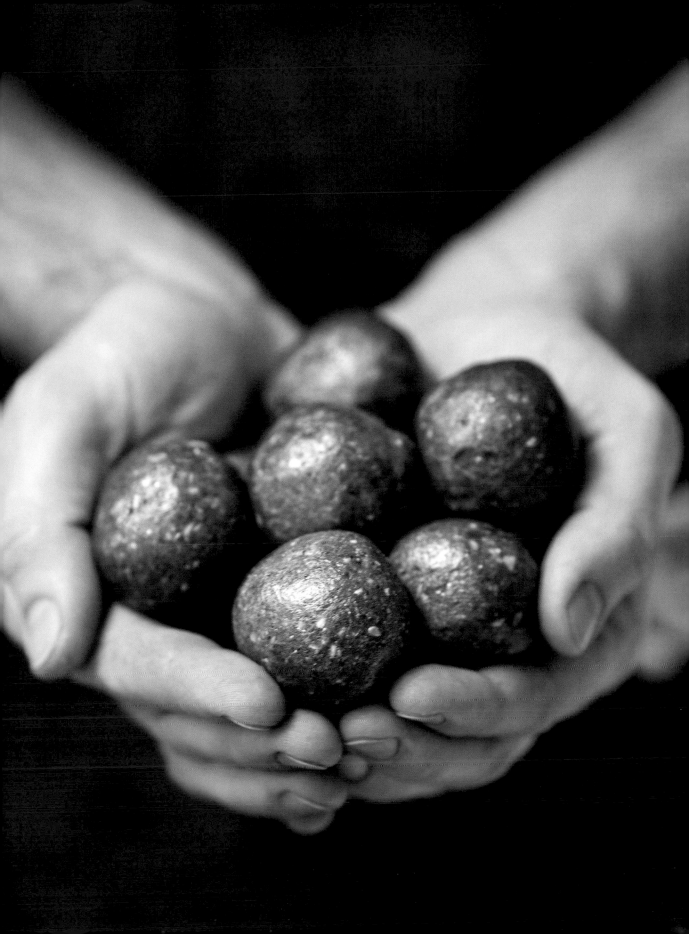

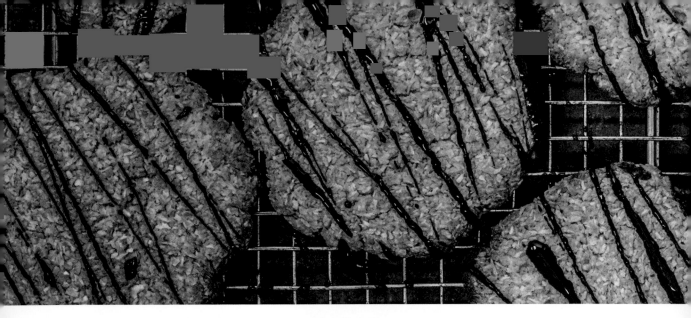

COCONUT + CHOCOLATE BISCUITS

THERE IS NO OTHER WAY TO DESCRIBE THESE THAN A BIT OF AN AWESOME TREAT – THEY TASTE AMAZING!

MAKES 12

125g rolled oats
100g desiccated coconut
50g ground almonds
3 tablespoons runny honey
2 tablespoons coconut oil
1 teaspoon coconut extract or almond extract
Pinch of fine sea salt
1 large free-range egg
1 large free-range egg white

TO DECORATE

75g dark chocolate (70% cocoa solids)

PER BISCUIT:
KCAL: 168 **FAT:** 11g
CARBS: 12g **PROTEIN:** 4g

Preheat the oven to 160°C/gas mark 3 and line two baking sheets with baking parchment.

Blend the oats in a food processor for 2 minutes until you have a coarse powder. Add the remaining ingredients and pulse until the mixture comes together to form a rough ball. Roll into 12 equal balls then space out evenly on the lined trays. Squash the rounds down with your fingertips to make 5mm-thick discs, then bake for 15 minutes until golden.

Meanwhile, break the chocolate into small pieces into a heatproof bowl. Microwave on medium power for 30 seconds then stir. Heat in 30-second bursts (it'll take 2 or 3 bursts, depending on the strength of your microwave) until the chocolate has just melted; chocolate can burn easily so be careful not to overheat it. (Alternatively, set the bowl over a pan of simmering water and stir until liquid.)

Transfer the biscuits to a wire rack to cool completely, then drizzle with the melted chocolate. Leave to set.

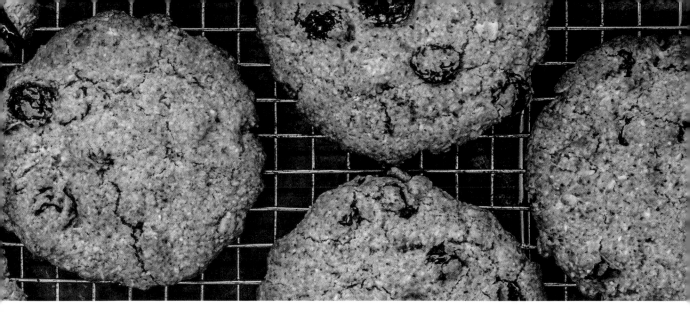

OATMEAL RAISIN COOKIES

EVERYONE LOVES A GOOD COOKIE, RIGHT? THESE ARE SERIOUSLY GOOOOD! THEY MAKE A GREAT SNACK FOR YOUR DAY BUT YOU COULD ALSO SERVE THESE AS AN ALTERNATIVE TO DESSERT.

MAKES 12

250g rolled oats
120g raisins
1½ teaspoons baking powder
1½ teaspoons ground cinnamon
¼ teaspoon salt
120ml runny honey
4 tablespoons coconut oil, melted
1 large free-range egg
1 teaspoon vanilla extract

Preheat the oven to 180°C/gas mark 4 and line two baking sheets with baking parchment.

Pour 150g of the oats into a food processor and blend to a fine powder. Pour the blended oats into a large bowl and stir in the remaining oats, the raisins, baking powder, cinnamon and salt. Whisk together the honey, coconut oil, egg and vanilla extract in a jug then pour into the bowl with the dry ingredients.

Stir to combine then drop heaped tablespoons of the cookie dough onto the lined baking trays, leaving a gap of at least 5cm between each one as they will spread during cooking. Use wet fingers to flatten the dough slightly then bake for 10 minutes until golden brown and crisp around the edges. Leave to cool on the baking sheets for 10 minutes then transfer to a wire rack to cool completely.

PER COOKIE:
KCAL: 207   FAT: 7g
CARBS: 32g   PROTEIN: 4g

BETTER

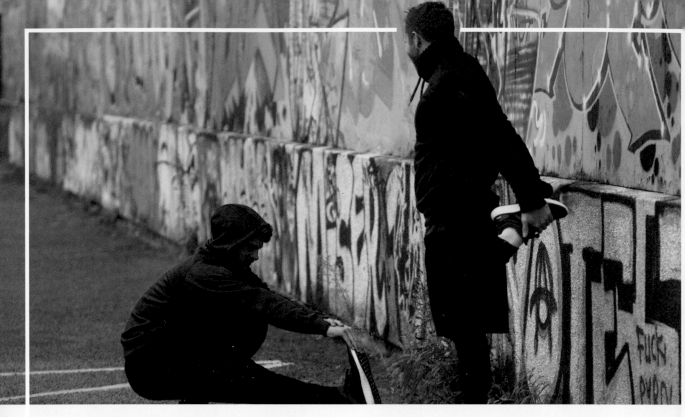

This chapter is all about getting you moving and, most importantly, doing it right. Exercise isn't as simple as just getting into the gym and pushing yourself until you can't breathe. It's about so much more than that and we want to arm you with all the necessary techniques to help you achieve your goals.

First, you need to ask yourself the right questions. Why do I train? What is my goal? Do I need to update my goals? Do I need help? Am I enjoying my training?

The fitness industry has a great ability to overcomplicate things, but just as with the EAT WELL chapter, you need to work out what's best for you.

Exercise will be different for all of us. Some prefer lifting heavy weights, while others prefer yoga, for instance. Whatever you want

to do is up to you, but here we have constructed workout plans full of the moves we think are most important, with loads of photos to show you exactly how to do them – with little to no equipment. If you are a gym goer, don't worry; we have that covered, too, with progressive training plans to keep you going and test you along the way.

Remember, the energy deficit or surplus you create via your diet and training will ultimately dictate whether you gain weight or lose it. If your goal is to build muscle then you need to eat enough in conjunction with training. If your goal is fat loss you need to be in an energy deficit as well as training in the same manner. Be sure to go back to the EAT WELL chapter and adjust your TDEE, once you have decided on your workout regime.

WHY SHOULD I TRAIN?

Aside from burning calories, working out has so many benefits. You'll improve your bone density and strength to name a few. Training will also have a great effect on your overall mood.

Unfortunately, we are led to believe that it only takes a matter of weeks to completely change your body into magazine cover model material. For a few people who are already in great shape,

this might be the case, but for most of us this just isn't realistic.

The plans and techniques we are going to show you can change your body. Aimed at beginner, intermediate and advanced readers, all the tools you need to get in shape and achieve your goals are right here.

ASK YOURSELF

Once you have your goal in mind, be it fat loss or muscle gain, you need to make sure that you have what it takes to stick to it by asking some questions:

Is this what I really want?
How long will it take me to achieve it?
What will achieving this give me?
Can I see myself doing this in
eight weeks' time?

When it comes down to it you're the only person who has to put yourself through the workouts; we believe the only true way to stay motivated long term is by setting goals selfishly and honestly for no one but yourself. It's also very important to remember that not everyone trains purely to 'look great'. So many people train just for health, as a hobby or just to sweat it out a little every now and again, so please never feel pressured to make your goal an

aesthetic one. Training is purely what you want it to be.

Remember: this is a lifestyle change, not a race.

A great way to make sure that you're going to stick to your chosen plan is to make sure you can fit it into your life. Write down all of the commitments you already have and how much time they take up. Oh, and remember to factor in time for sleep: you'd be surprised at how many people forget that they need to sleep when motivation takes hold! Then you won't have any excuses to miss a workout.

Remember, if your goal is fat loss and you are losing 1lb a week, you are doing great; if you want to gain muscle then aim for ¼–½lb a week. These are realistic results, although hard to track in the long term.

WURKOUTS

CARDIOVASCULAR EXERCISE

Cardio is like Marmite – you either love it or you hate it! Either way, it serves a purpose: regular cardio will reduce your resting heart rate, improve your fitness and burn extra calories – thus helping you to lose more fat. There are many different ways to improve your cardiovascular fitness and it's not limited to the treadmill. You can swim, bike, go for walks or runs, or play your favourite sport. It simply comes down to execution.

HIIT

This stands for High Intensity Interval Training, and we are big fans. It has the benefit of taking less time than, say, a jog, but it requires you to work your butt off for 10–20 minutes at a near-maximum level. You can do treadmill work with 20-second sprints and 40 seconds recovery, or just use your body weight with circuit exercises such as burpees and jump lunges. It's so versatile, the options are endless, and you will burn tons of calories. Even after your HIIT session has finished, you have the potential to still be burning calories for a prolonged period of time.

PROGRESSIVE OVERLOAD

This is the most important rule of progression. You have to keep changing and progressing the stimulus: whether it's the weight you lift, the number of reps you complete, the metres you run or the amount of time you do it in. When you first start exercising you improve faster than those who have been training for a year or so – this is known as beginner gains. Basically, your body is learning to innovate more motor units or muscle fibres and neurons and the more motor units you innovate the more force you can produce.

WHEN SHOULD I TRAIN?

There is no such thing as the 'best time' to train. It comes down to you, your lifestyle and your preference. This may sound like a dodge by us, but let us explain: if you're not a morning person why force yourself to get up even earlier to train? Just do it later. It really is that simple. If you pick a time that's good for you, you'll work much harder and you will be much more likely to stick at it long term. It may take a few weeks of trial and error to find the best workout time for you, but remember to give each method a chance for a few weeks before changing it.

> WHEN WE START SOMETHING NEW, WE ALWAYS FIND IT TOUGH, BUT THE AWESOME FEELING THAT FOLLOWS MAKES IT ALL SO WORTHWHILE.

We have included plans with step-by-step moves for home, gym and HIIT workouts. Please remember to be careful, and don't try anything too difficult straight away as we are trained professionals, and some of the moves can be dangerous if you're not as used to them as we are. We couldn't photograph every single move we've mentioned, but we've made sure that beginners training from home has everything explained here.

BEGINNER

IF YOU'RE COMPLETELY NEW TO TRAINING OR USING ANY FORM OF RESISTANCE IN YOUR WORKOUTS, THIS PLAN WILL BE THE PERFECT PLACE FOR YOU TO START. YOU CAN USE IT IN THE GYM OR AT HOME. THERE ARE PLENTY OF MOVE BETTER ANNOTATED PICTURES FOR YOU TO LOOK THROUGH TO MAKE SURE YOU'RE DOING THE MOVES CORRECTLY. IT STARTS WITH A THREE-DAY WORKOUT WEEK, COVERING ALL YOUR MAJOR MUSCLE GROUPS AND MOVES TO HELP GET YOUR BODY USED TO RESISTANCE TRAINING, GAIN SOME STRENGTH AND KEEP YOUR GOALS ON TRACK.

INTERMEDIATE

THIS IS FOR THE GUYS AND GIRLS AMONG YOU WHO'VE ALREADY TRAINED FOR A WHILE, OR HAVE PAST GYM EXPERIENCE, SO YOU KNOW YOUR WAY AROUND A WORKOUT. THIS IS A PROGRESSIVE PLAN THAT WILL DEFINITELY TEST YOU AND KEEP YOUR BODY GUESSING. SOME OF THESE MOVES ARE ILLUSTRATED.

ADVANCED

FOR THE GYM BUNNIES OUT THERE. YOU ARE ALREADY COMFORTABLE IN THE GYM AND FREE WEIGHTS SECTION AND USED TO TRAINING THREE TO FIVE DAYS A WEEK. THESE PLANS ARE GOING TO GET TOUGH, MIXING UP REP RANGES, STYLES AND TEMPOS TO GET MORE FOCUS ON THE MUSCLE GROUPS BEING WORKED. A FEW OF THESE MOVES ARE ILLUSTRATED.

THE ⑤ MOST COMMON TRAINING QUESTIONS

① WHAT ARE REPS AND SETS?

Reps and sets create the structure of your workout. A rep (or repetition) is one completed movement, so one squat, for instance. Once you have gone all the way down to your range in a squat and returned to your start position you have then completed one rep! A set is the number of reps you do without stopping. So again, with a squat, if you decide to do ten squats then stop, that's one set.

② HOW CAN I LOSE THIS LAST BIT OF FAT AROUND MY TUMMY?

That last bit of fat that hangs around is normally the hardest to get rid of because we cannot spot reduce fat. Doing lots of sit-ups will not help – in fact you will be wasting your time as you could be using it to perform exercises that burn many more calories. Quite simply, that last bit of body fat requires you to keep going and potentially create more of a caloric deficit; that's why it's hard, because it requires more effort.

③ SHOULD I SQUAT AS LOW AS I CAN?

The first thing to understand with squats is that they are a skill, so the more you do them the better you will become. If you have the flexibility and skill then yes, going low enough so that your hips are lower than your knees is ideal as it has a bigger range of motion and will recruit more muscles in the exercise. However, if you lack the flexibility and skill you will compromise your technique and increase the risk of injury, especially when lifting heavy weights. If this is the case, then work on your tight areas – these are usually the ankles, calves, hamstrings and hip flexors, as well as mid to upper back.

④ HOW OFTEN SHOULD I TRAIN?

To achieve real change in your physique and your performance, we suggest you train three to five times per week for forty to sixty minutes. If you feel you can recover in time you can do more, but beware of overdoing it. We suggest that you take one week in every six to eight and train at about forty per cent of your usual rate, to rest but also to keep your motor units from slacking. This is called a De-load Week.

⑤ WHY CAN'T I BUILD MUSCLE?

This one is quite simple. Either you are not eating enough or you are not training effectively. Building muscle requires you to push your body further than it has been before, followed by getting adequate rest and recovery.

RULES TO REMEMBER:

- Train for yourself, with your own reasons and goals in mind.
- Stop, rest and assess every six to eight weeks to make sure you're on track.
- Balance is key: don't devote your life to the gym. Train hard, recover harder!
- If you are ever unsure of how to do something, ask an experienced coach. Do remember that we will be here every single step of the way, and you can always reach out to us on any of our social media platforms.

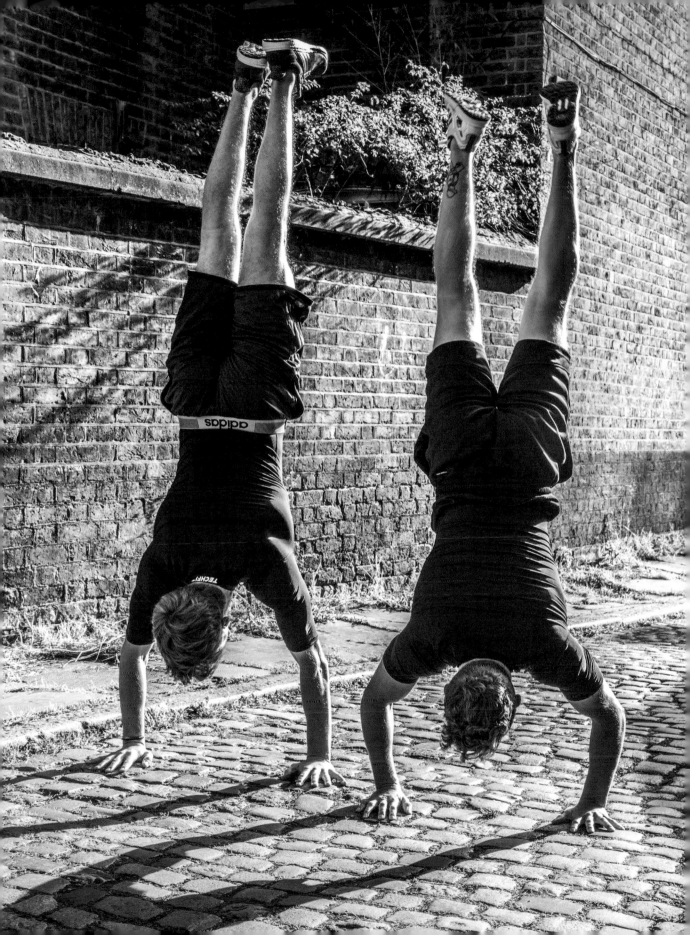

BEGINNER
HOME PLAN

DAY 1 - COMPLETE 10 MIN WARM-UP FIRST*	REPS	SETS	REST
1A SQUATS	30	3	
1B LUNGES	10 each leg	3	1 min
2A HIGH KNEES	30s	3	
2B SQUAT HOLD	30s	3	1 min
3A PUSH UPS (KNEEL IF NEEDED)	10 reps	3	
3B MOUNTAIN CLIMBERS	10 reps	3	1 min
4A PLANK HOLD	30s	3	
4B SQUAT THRUSTS	30s	3	1 min
5A GLUTE BRIDGE	30	3	
5B REVERSE MOUNTAIN CLIMBERS	20	3	1 min

DAY 2 - COMPLETE 10 MIN WARM-UP FIRST*	REPS	SETS	REST
CHALLENGE DAY, INVERSE LADDERS:			
SQUATS	15-1		
ALTERNATING LUNGES	15-1		
SQUAT THRUSTS	15-1		
PUSH UPS	15-1		
WALK DOWNS	15-1		
MOUNTAIN CLIMBERS	15-1		

The goal of inverse ladders is to finish the ladder in your fastest time possible, start by doing 15 of each exercise then 14,13,12,11 and so on until you reach 1. Aim for as little rest as possible!

On this beginner plan we are aiming to build some fundamental strength, flexibility, coordination and burn lots of calories and thus fat. You may find you cannot do some exercises; if that is the case there are always easier alternatives for you to progress from. If you really need a longer rest than stated take it, but do your best to push yourself during each workout. Where you see exercises labelled, e.g. 1A, 2B etc, these are 'superset' moves, which need to be completed back to back without taking a rest.

DAY 3 - COMPLETE 10 MIN WARM-UP FIRST*	REPS	3	REST
1A HIGH KNEES	30s	3	
1B BULGARIAN SPLIT SQUAT	10 each leg	3	1 min
2A SQUAT JUMPS	20	3	
2B SQUAT THRUSTS	30	3	1 min
3A MOUNTAIN CLIMBERS	30	3	
3B CURTSY LUNGES	20 each leg	3	1 min
4A BURPEES (NO JUMP)	10	3	
4B PRONE BACK EXTENSION	20	3	1 min
5 SPIDERMAN PLANK CRUNCH	15 each side	3	30 sec

*A warm-up is a dynamic pulse raiser: anything that brings the heart rate up gradually, gets the blood pumping, and lubricates the joints ready to train. For example: a walk, a slow jog around the block, or some simple squats, lunges and body rotations.

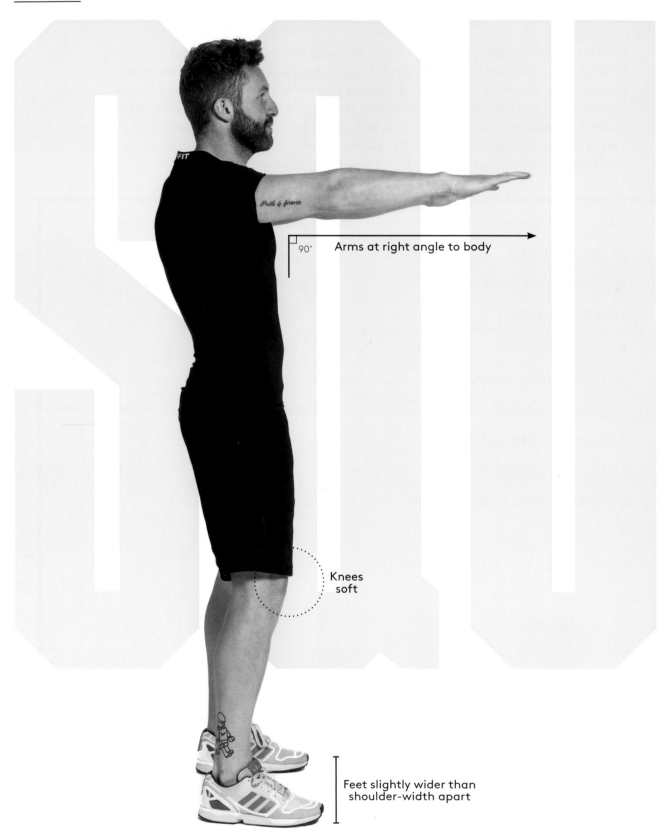

90°

Arms at right angle to body

Knees
soft

Feet slightly wider than
shoulder-width apart

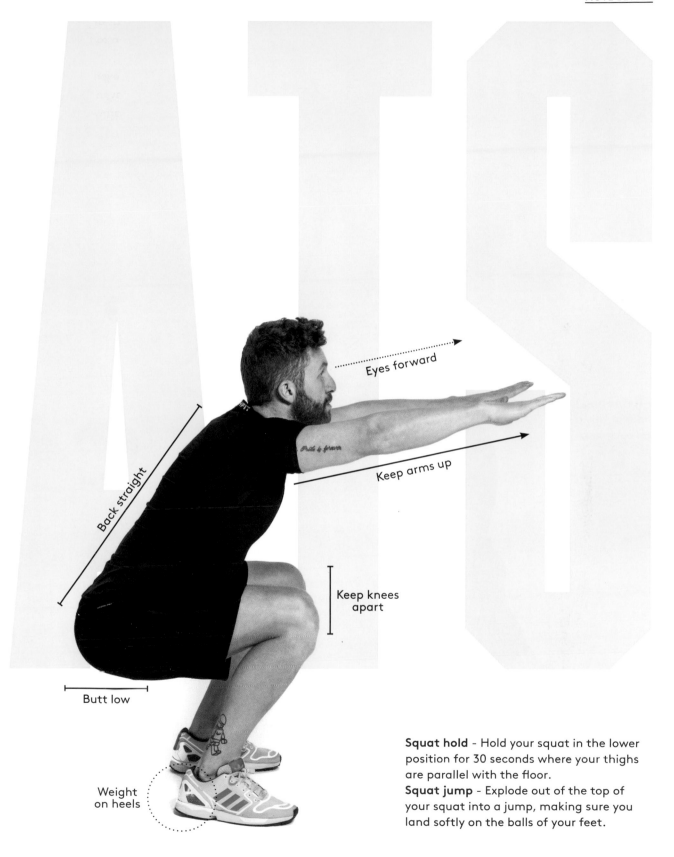

Eyes forward

Back straight

Keep arms up

Keep knees apart

Butt low

Weight on heels

Squat hold - Hold your squat in the lower position for 30 seconds where your thighs are parallel with the floor.

Squat jump - Explode out of the top of your squat into a jump, making sure you land softly on the balls of your feet.

LUNGES

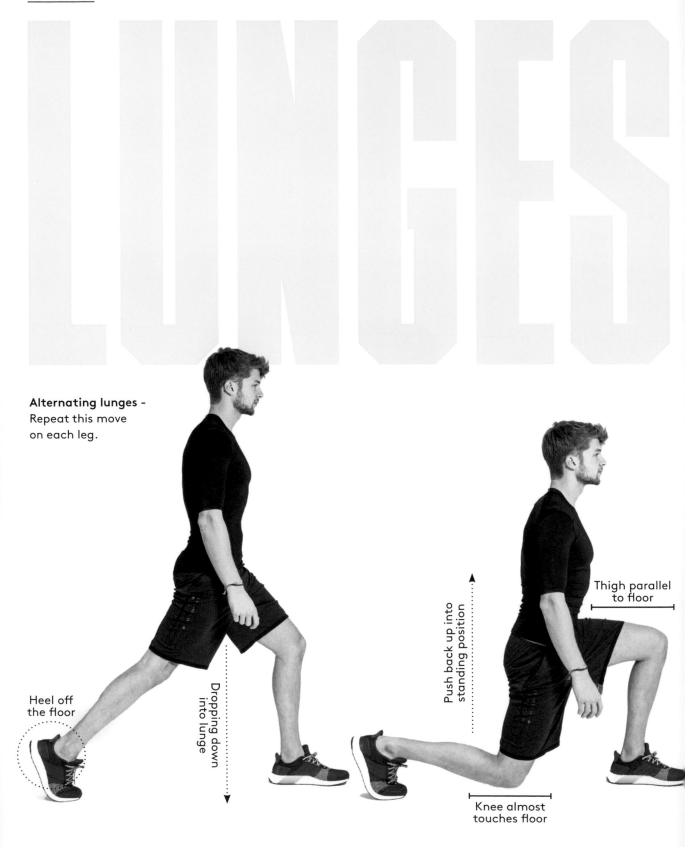

Alternating lunges -
Repeat this move
on each leg.

Heel off
the floor

Dropping down
into lunge

Push back up into
standing position

Thigh parallel
to floor

Knee almost
touches floor

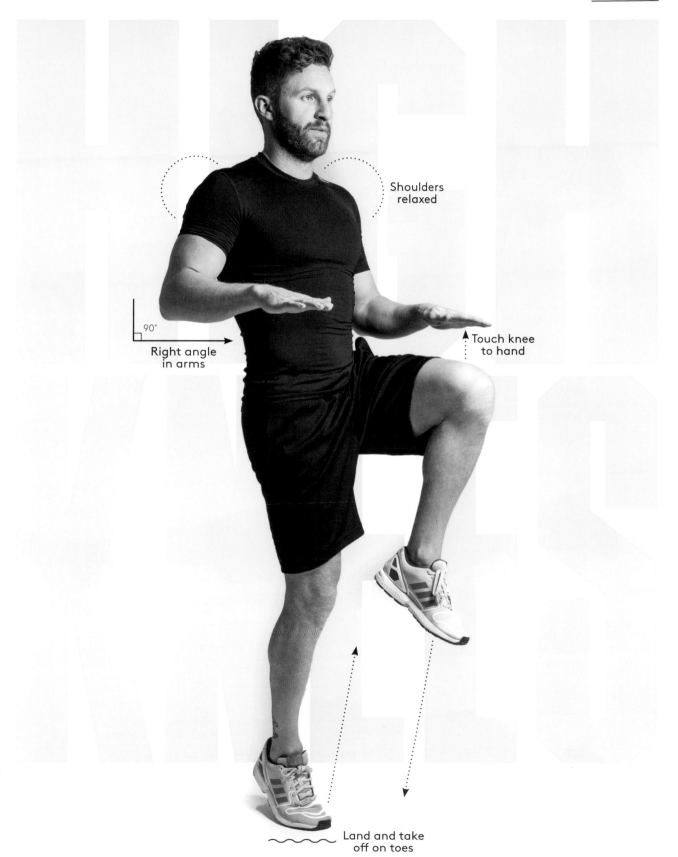

Shoulders
relaxed

90°

Right angle
in arms

Touch knee
to hand

Land and take
off on toes

PUSH UPS

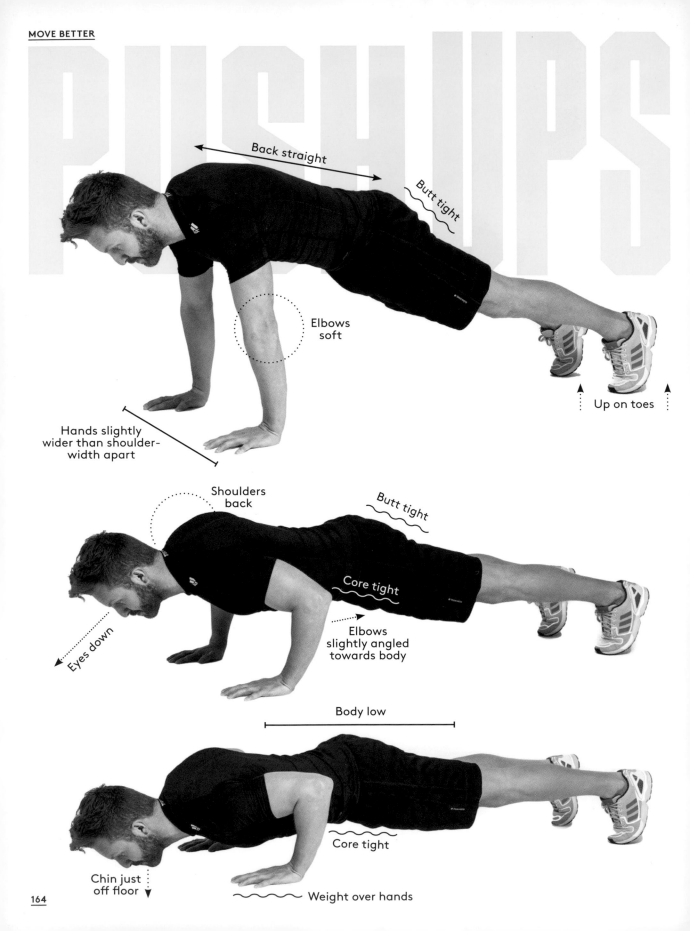

Back straight

Butt tight

Elbows soft

Up on toes

Hands slightly wider than shoulder-width apart

Shoulders back

Butt tight

Core tight

Eyes down

Elbows slightly angled towards body

Body low

Core tight

Chin just off floor

Weight over hands

PLANK HOLD

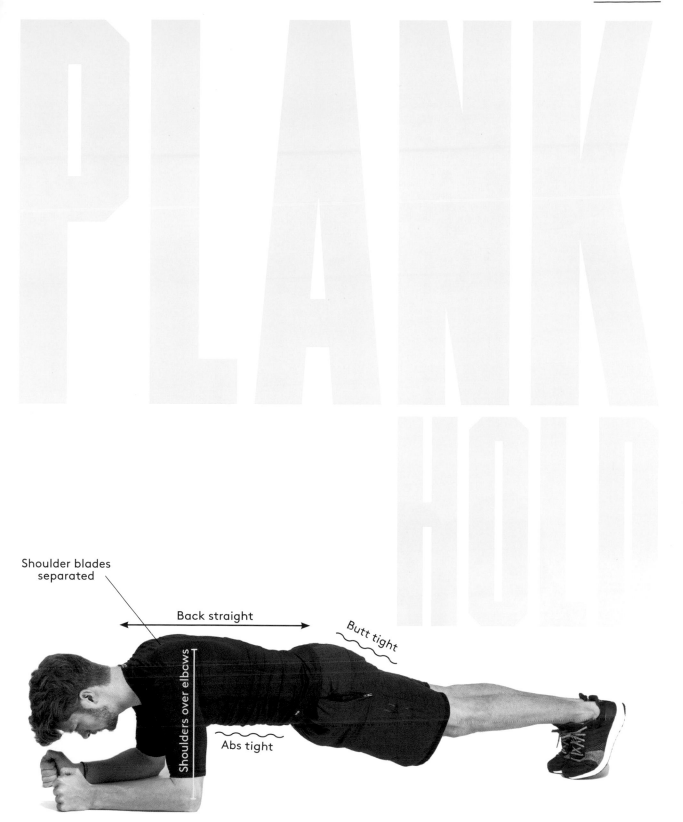

Shoulder blades separated

Back straight

Butt tight

Shoulders over elbows

Abs tight

SQUAT THRUSTS

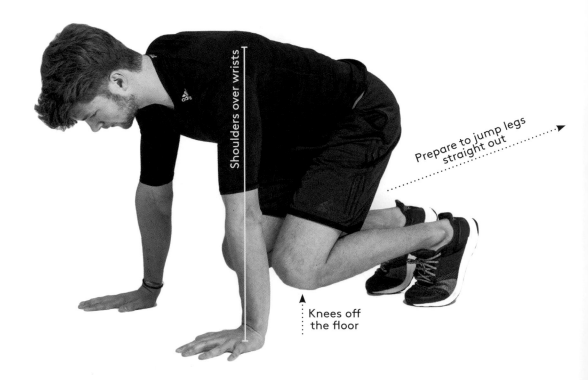

Shoulders over wrists

Prepare to jump legs straight out

Knees off the floor

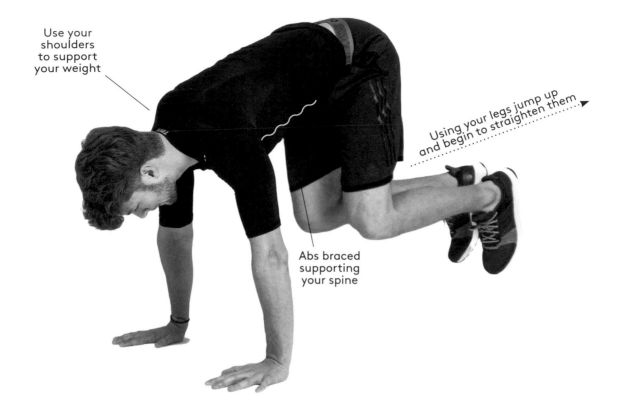

Use your shoulders to support your weight

Using your legs jump up and begin to straighten them

Abs braced supporting your spine

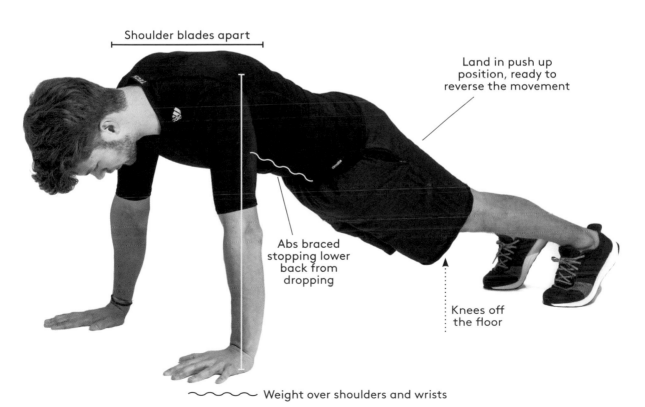

Shoulder blades apart

Land in push up position, ready to reverse the movement

Abs braced stopping lower back from dropping

Knees off the floor

Weight over shoulders and wrists

GLUTE BRIDGE

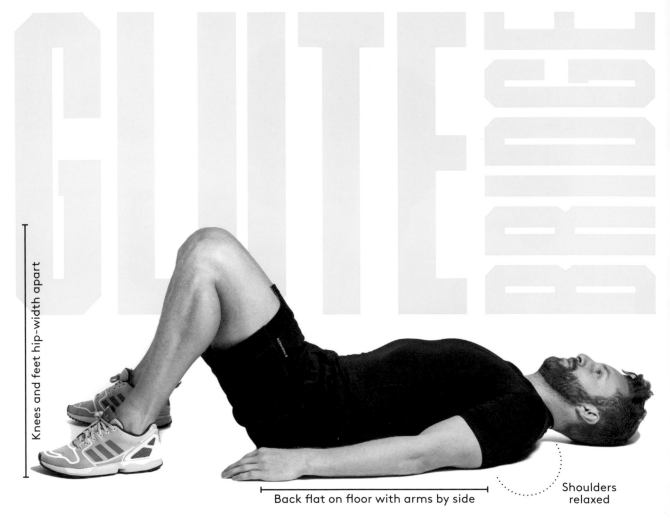

Knees and feet hip-width apart

Back flat on floor with arms by side

Shoulders relaxed

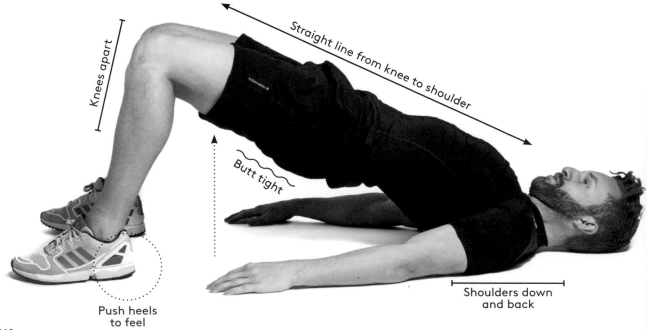

Knees apart

Straight line from knee to shoulder

Butt tight

Push heels to feel

Shoulders down and back

MOUNTAIN CLIMBERS

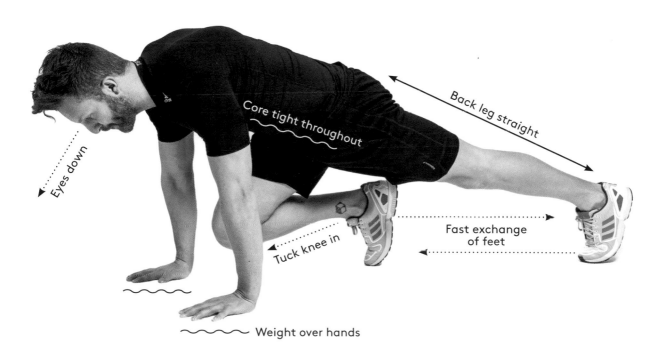

Back leg straight

Core tight throughout

Eyes down

Tuck knee in

Fast exchange of feet

Weight over hands

REVERSE MOUNTAIN

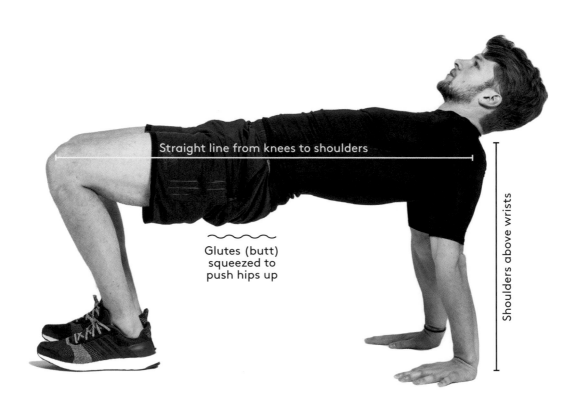

Straight line from knees to shoulders

Glutes (butt) squeezed to push hips up

Shoulders above wrists

CLIMBERS

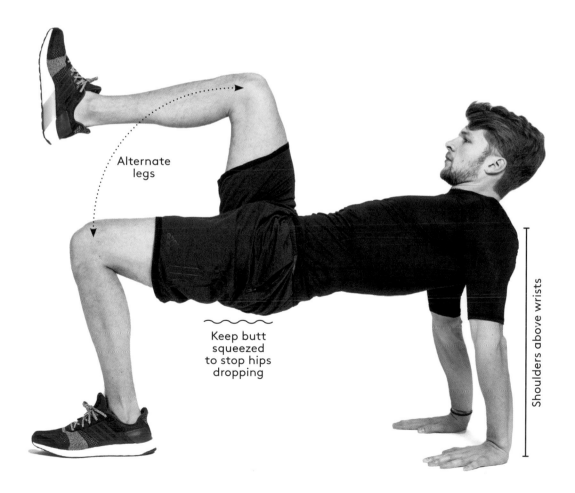

Alternate legs

Keep butt squeezed to stop hips dropping

Shoulders above wrists

WALK

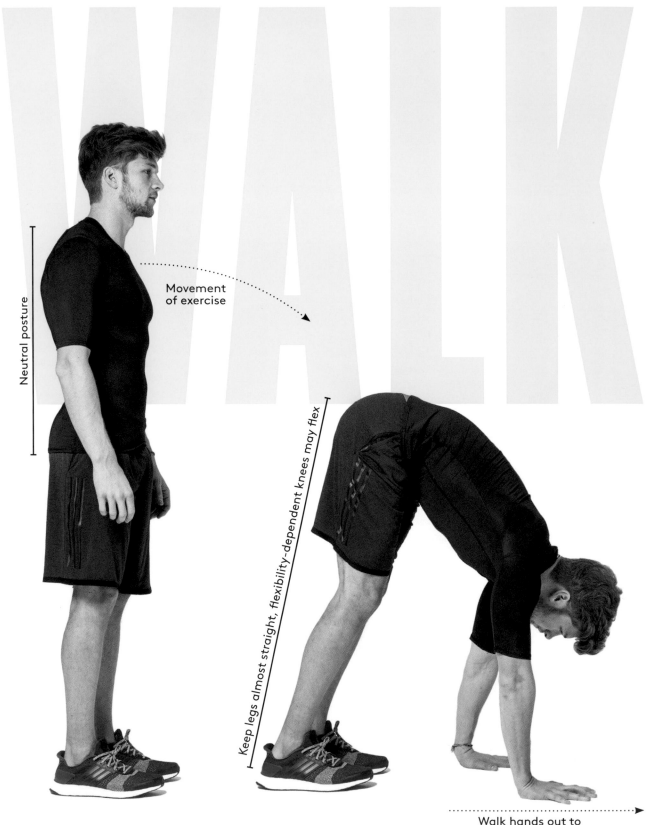

Neutral posture

Movement of exercise

Keep legs almost straight, flexibility-dependent knees may flex

Walk hands out to push up position

DOWNS

Back straight

Abs braced

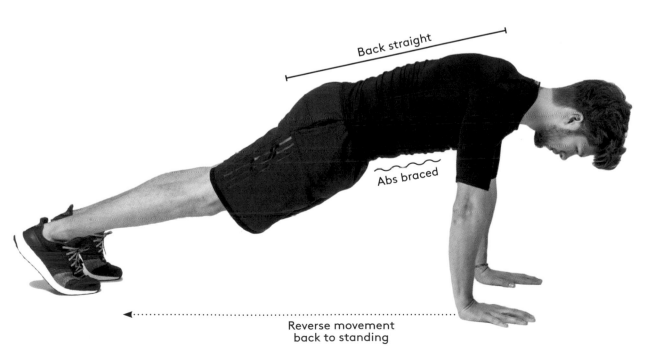

Reverse movement
back to standing

BULGARIAN

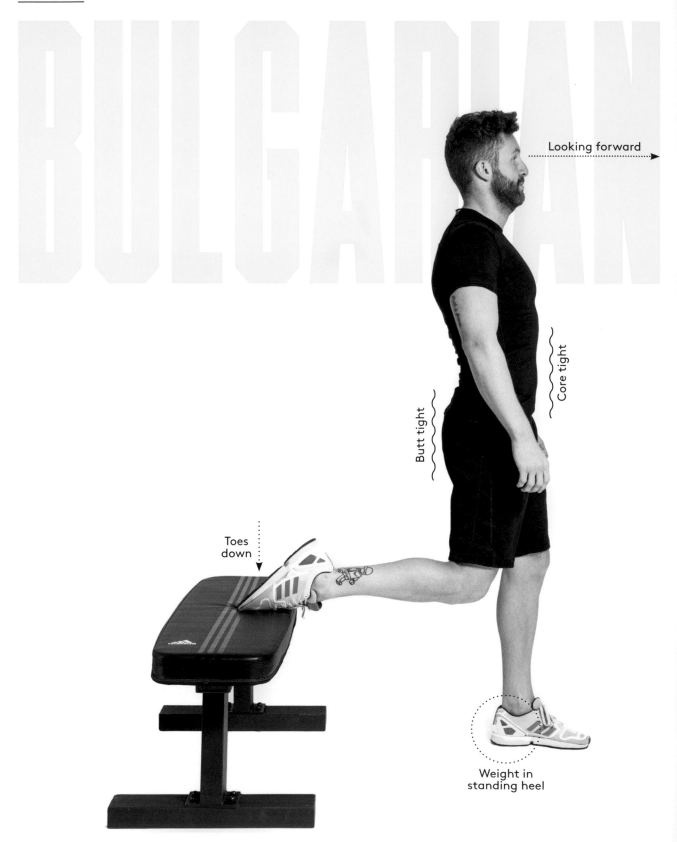

Looking forward

Core tight

Butt tight

Toes down

Weight in standing heel

SPLIT SQUAT

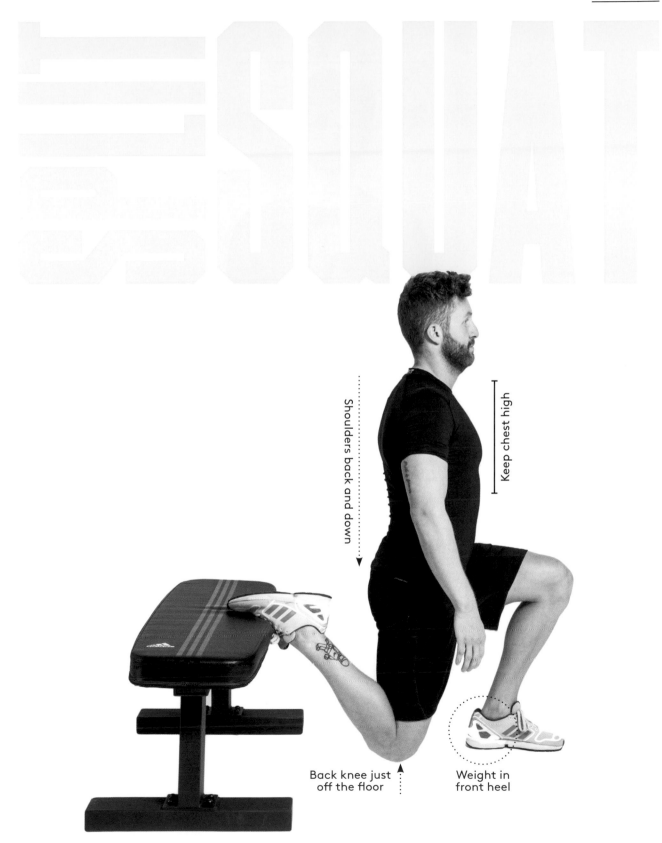

Keep chest high

Shoulders back and down

Back knee just off the floor

Weight in front heel

CURTSY

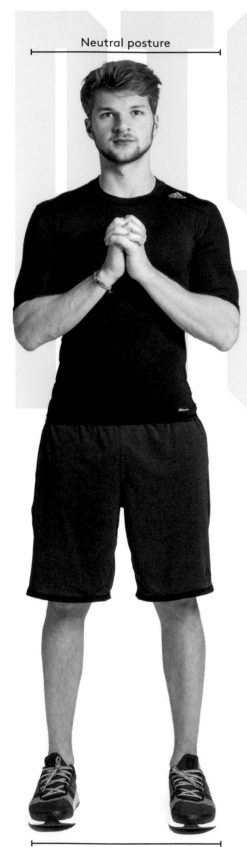

Neutral posture

Feet hip width apart

LUNGE

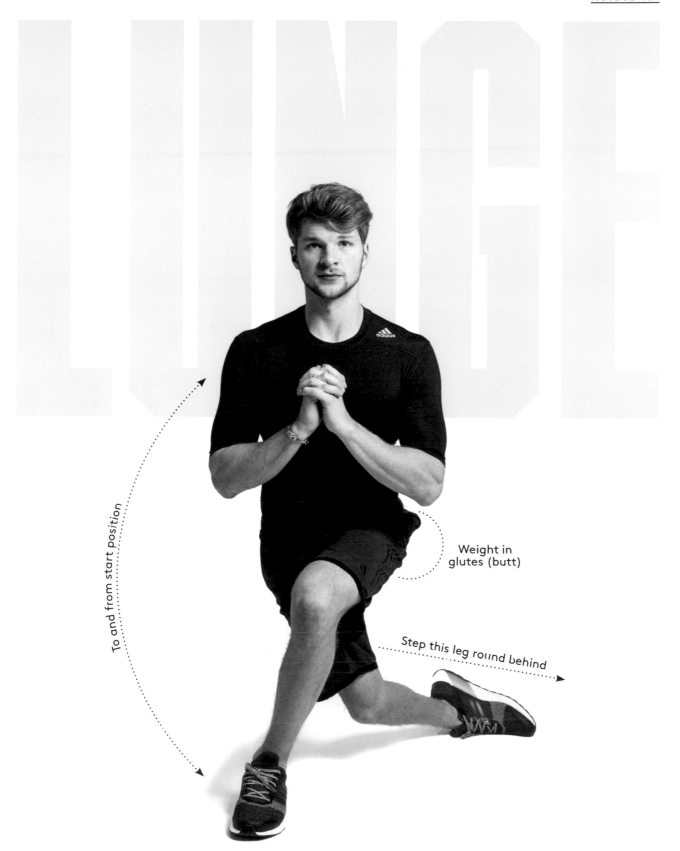

Weight in glutes (butt)

Step this leg round behind

To and from start position

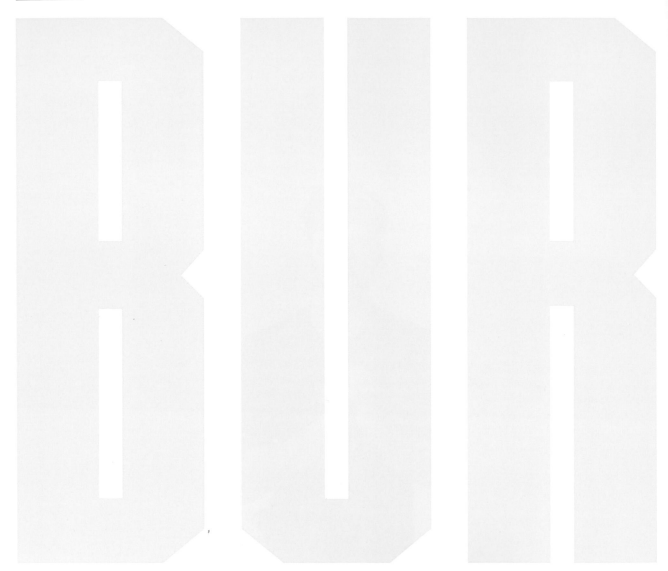

BUR

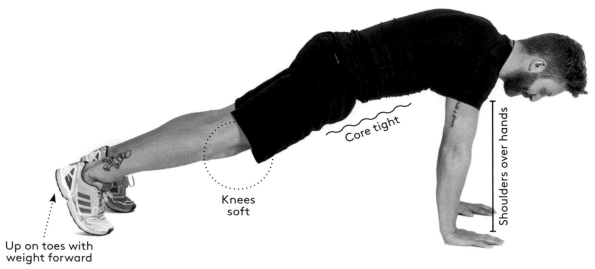

Core tight

Shoulders over hands

Knees soft

Up on toes with weight forward

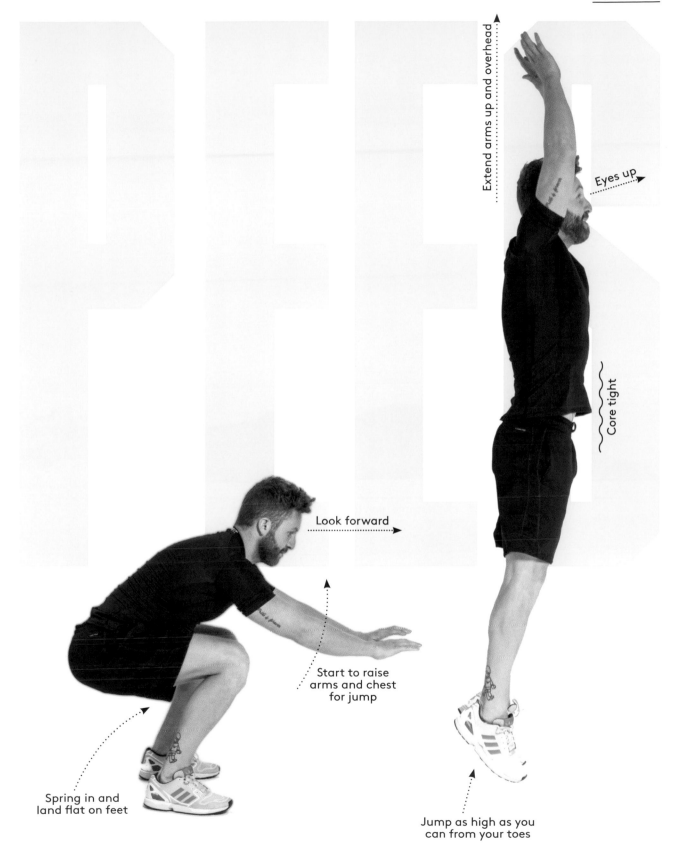

Extend arms up and overhead

Eyes up

Core tight

Look forward

Start to raise arms and chest for jump

Spring in and land flat on feet

Jump as high as you can from your toes

PRONE BACK EXTENSION

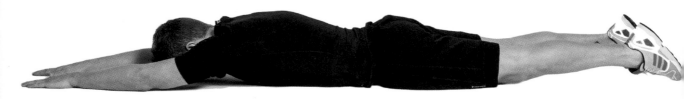

Simple, just lay flat and stretch out

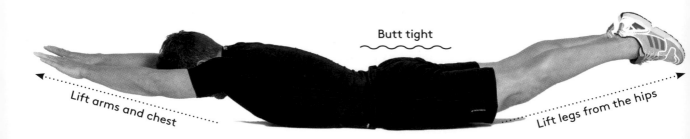

Butt tight

Lift arms and chest

Lift legs from the hips

SPIDERMAN PLANK CRUNCH

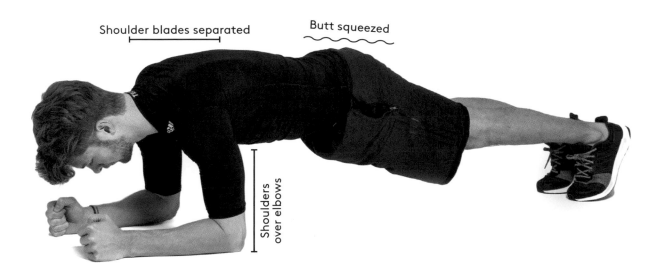

Shoulder blades separated

Butt squeezed

Shoulders over elbows

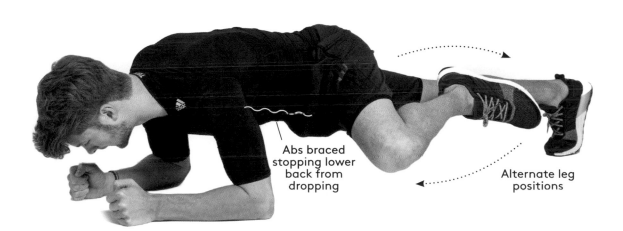

Abs braced stopping lower back from dropping

Alternate leg positions

INTERMEDIATE
HOME PLAN

DAY 1 - LEGS - COMPLETE 10 MIN WARM-UP FIRST*	REPS	SETS	REST
1A SINGLE LEX BOX SQUATS	12 each leg	3	
1B JUMP SQUATS	20	3	1 min
2A DUMBBELL WALKING LUNGES OR JUMP SPLIT LUNGES	20	3	
2B DRAG HAMSTRING CURL	15	3	1 min
3A KETTLE BELL SWINGS OR GLUTE BRIDGE MARCH	20	3	
3B GOBLET SQUATS (WEIGHTED) OR SUMO SQUATS	20	3	1 min
4A ALTERNATING SUPERMAN PLANK	30 sec	3	
4B JIU JITSU WALK THROUGHS	10 each side	3	1 min
5A GLUTE BRIDGE (LAY DUMBBELL ON HIPS)	30	3	
5B REVERSE CURLS	20	3	1 min

DAY 2 - UPPER - COMPLETE 10 MIN WARM-UP FIRST*	REPS	SETS	REST
1A TIGER PUSH UPS	12	4	
1B PIKE PUSH UPS	12	4	1 min
2A CHIN UPS	Failure[†]	4	1 min
3A RENEGADE ROW (USE DUMBBELLS)	12	4	
3B BURPEES	12	4	1 min
4A PLANK WALK UP	30 sec	3	
4B DIPS	Failure[†]	3	1 min

* See page 159

The first thing you will notice with the Intermediate plan is the introduction of weights. Everyone is at different levels so find a weight that works for you. Please be careful and ask an expert for advice if you need to.

DAY 3 - CIRCUITS - COMPLETE 10 MIN WARM-UP FIRST*	REPS	SETS	REST
CHALLENGE DAY - INTERMEDIATE HOME HIGH INTENSITY CIRCUIT			
SEE PAGE 218			

DAY 4 - LEGS - COMPLETE 10 MIN WARM-UP FIRST*	REPS	SETS	REST
DUMBBELL SHOULDER CIRCUIT:			
1A DUMBBELL ROWS	12	3	
1B STANDING SHOULDER PRESS	12	3	
1C SIDE RAISE	15	3	
1D REAR DELT RAISE	15	3	1 min
SPRINTS OUTSIDE OR JOG:			
SPRINTS	20-30 sec	15 min total	1 min walk

† Failure is when you can no longer complete a repetition with good technique, as your muscles have fatigued.

SINGLE LEG

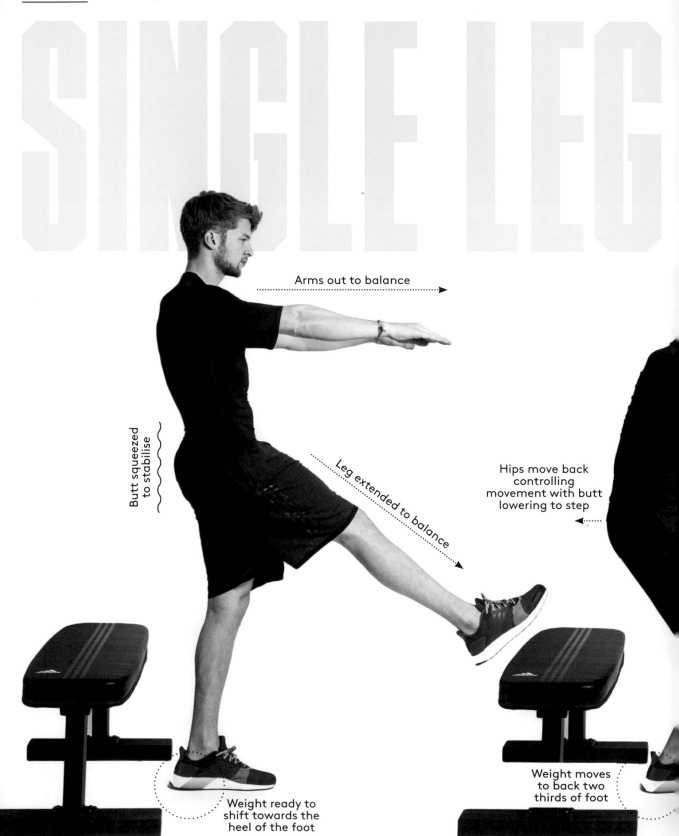

Arms out to balance →

Butt squeezed to stabilise

Leg extended to balance

Hips move back controlling movement with butt lowering to step

Weight ready to shift towards the heel of the foot

Weight moves to back two thirds of foot

BOX SQUATS

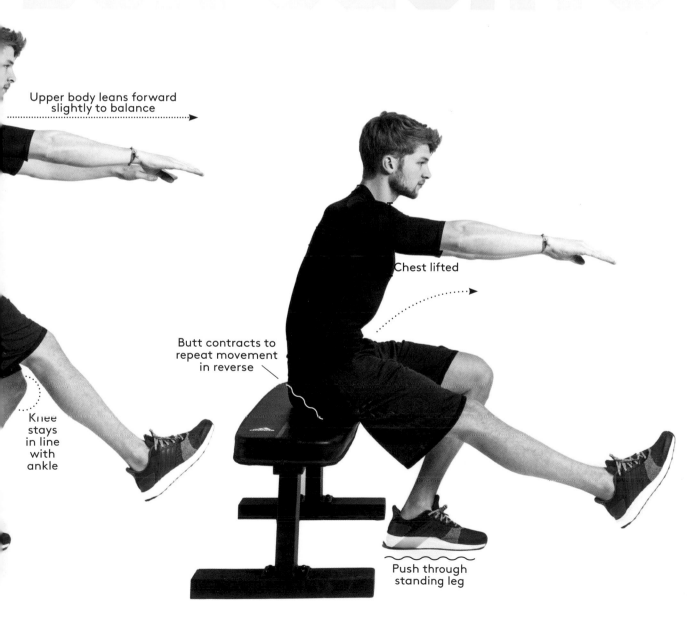

Upper body leans forward slightly to balance

Chest lifted

Butt contracts to repeat movement in reverse

Knee stays in line with ankle

Push through standing leg

DRAG HAMSTRING CURL

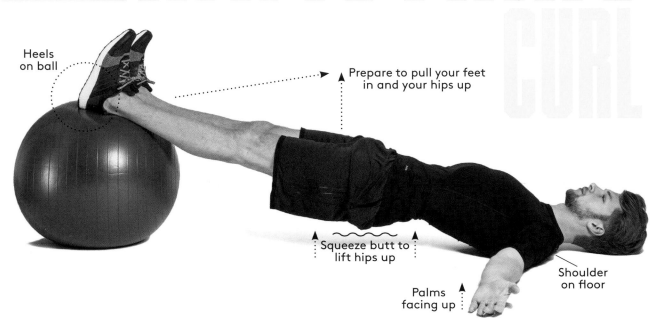

Heels on ball

Prepare to pull your feet in and your hips up

Squeeze butt to lift hips up

Palms facing up

Shoulder on floor

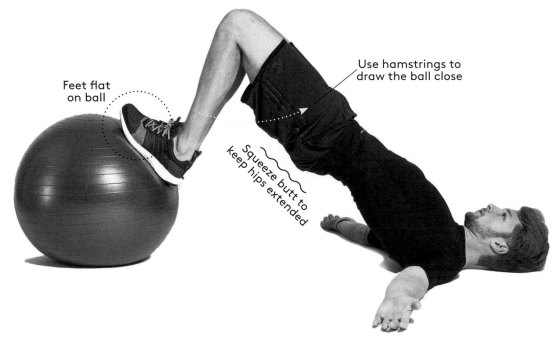

Feet flat on ball

Use hamstrings to draw the ball close

Squeeze butt to keep hips extended

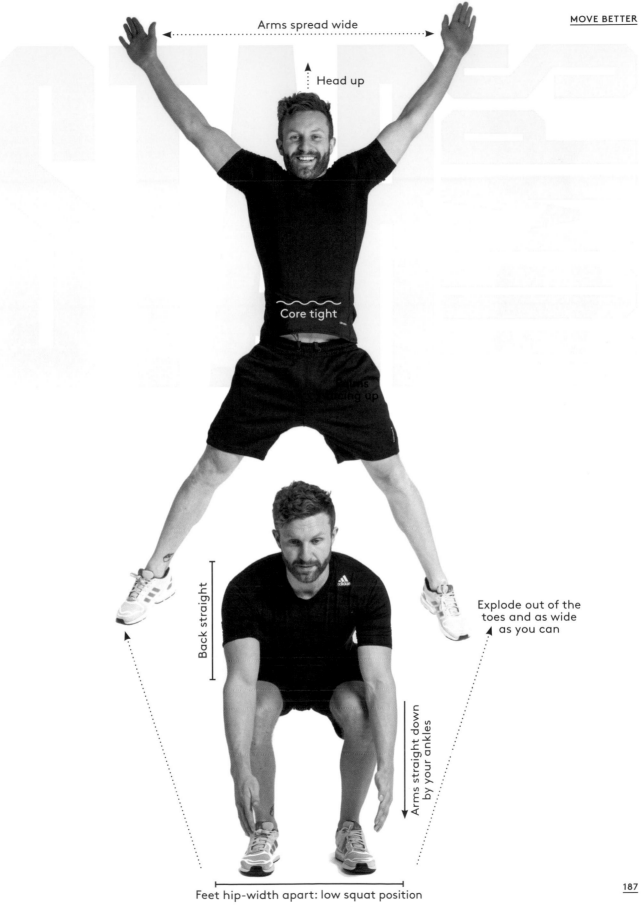

Arms spread wide

Head up

Core tight

Palms facing up

Back straight

Explode out of the toes and as wide as you can

Arms straight down by your ankles

Feet hip-width apart: low squat position

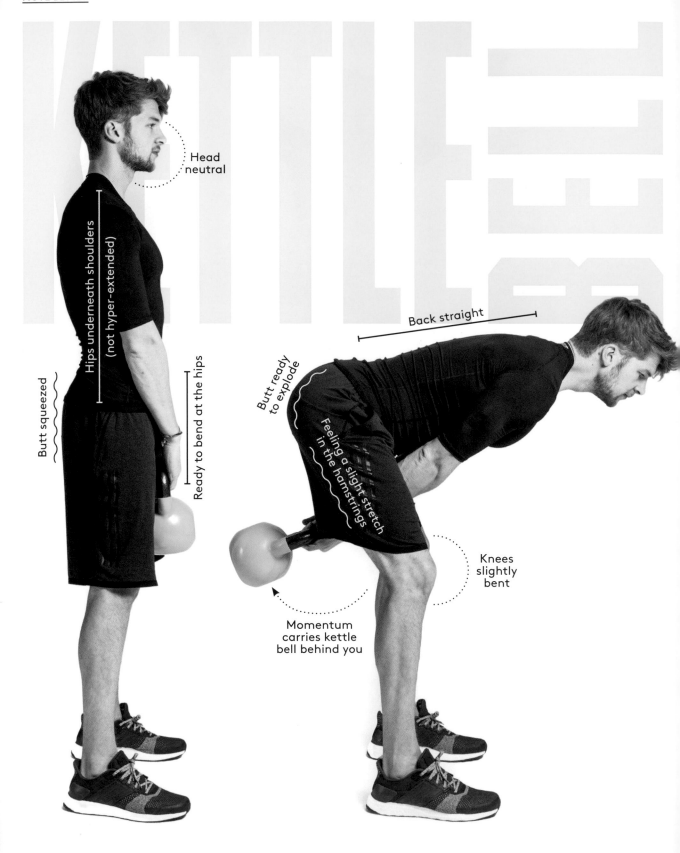

KETTLE BELL

Head neutral

Hips underneath shoulders (not hyper-extended)

Butt squeezed

Ready to bend at the hips

Back straight

Butt ready to explode

Feeling a slight stretch in the hamstrings

Knees slightly bent

Momentum carries kettle bell behind you

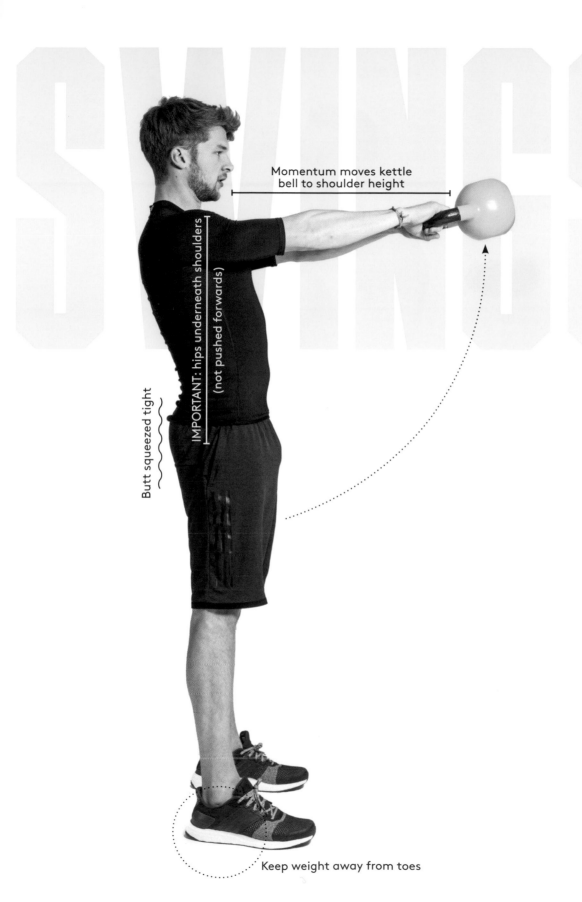

SWINGS

Momentum moves kettle bell to shoulder height

IMPORTANT: hips underneath shoulders (not pushed forwards)

Butt squeezed tight

Keep weight away from toes

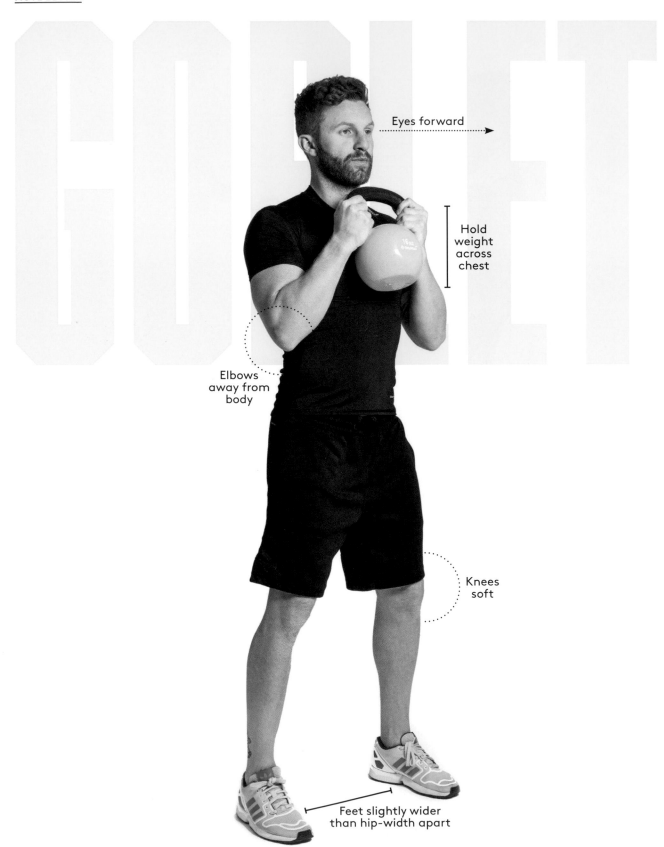

GOBLET

Eyes forward

Hold weight across chest

Elbows away from body

Knees soft

Feet slightly wider than hip-width apart

SQUATS

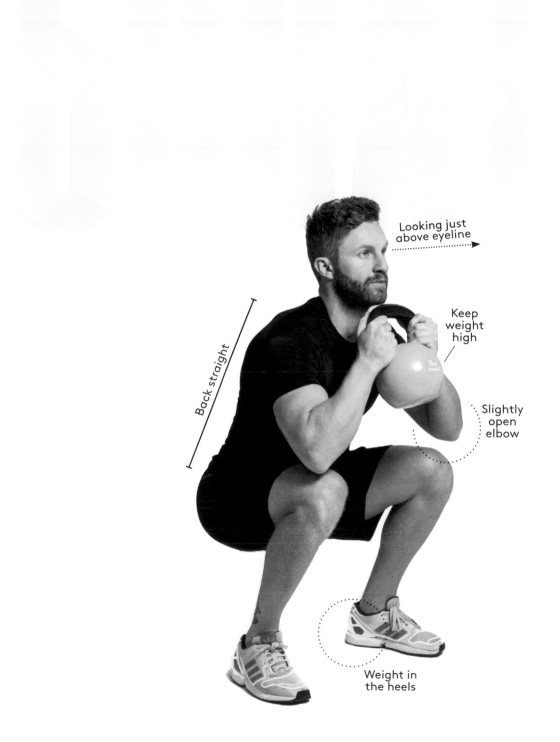

Looking just
above eyeline

Keep
weight
high

Back straight

Slightly
open
elbow

Weight in
the heels

JIU JITSU

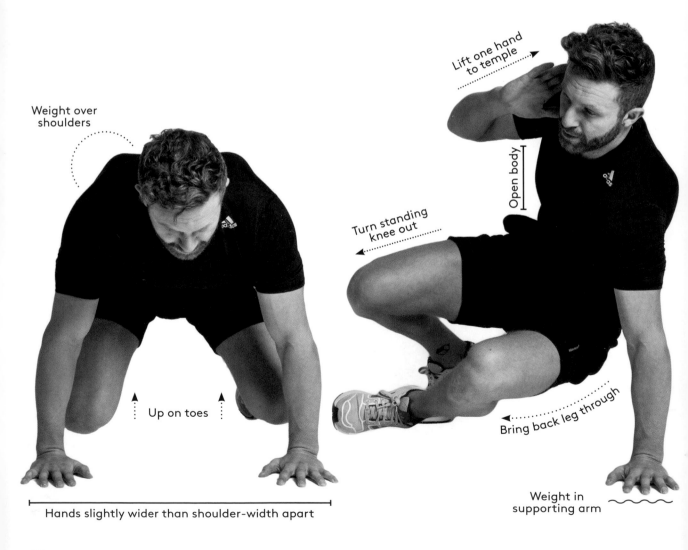

Weight over shoulders

Lift one hand to temple

Open body

Turn standing knee out

Bring back leg through

Up on toes

Weight in supporting arm

Hands slightly wider than shoulder-width apart

WALK THROUGHS

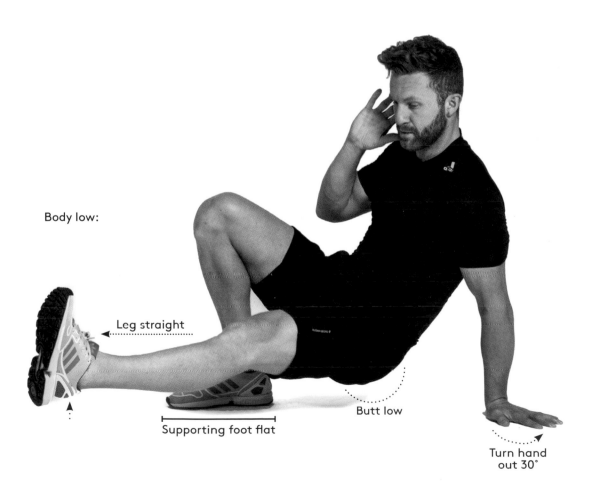

Body low:

Leg straight

Supporting foot flat

Butt low

Turn hand out 30°

WEIGHTED GLUTE BRIDGE

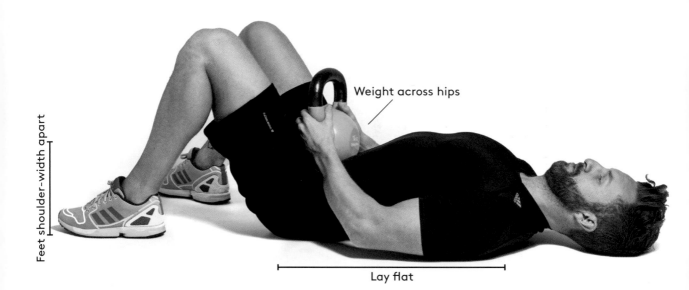

Feet shoulder-width apart

Weight across hips

Lay flat

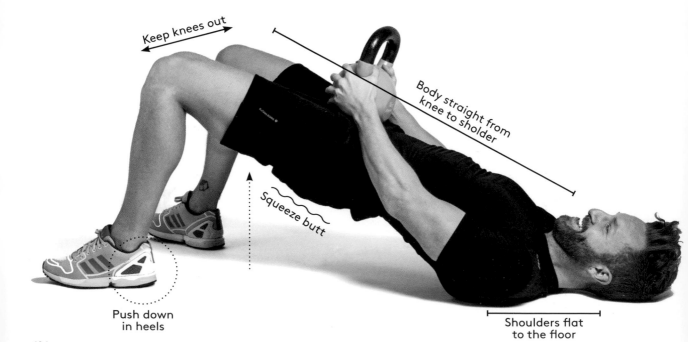

Keep knees out

Body straight from knee to sholder

Squeeze butt

Push down in heels

Shoulders flat to the floor

TIGER PUSH UPS

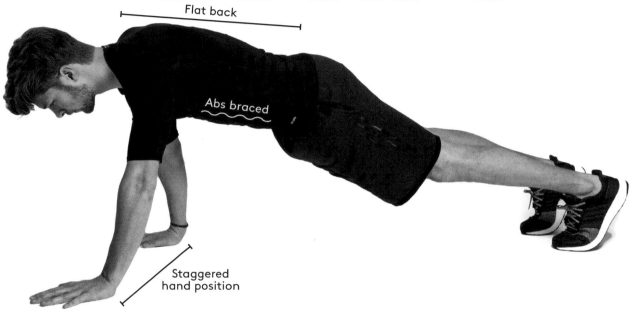

Flat back

Abs braced

Staggered
hand position

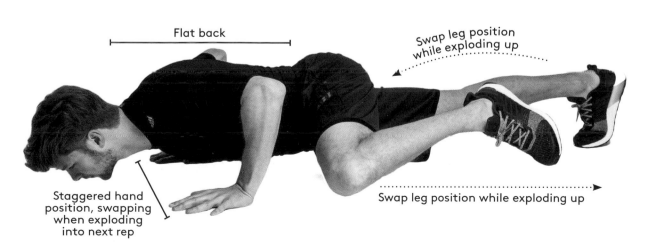

Flat back

Swap leg position
while exploding up

Staggered hand
position, swapping
when exploding
into next rep

Swap leg position while exploding up

PLANK

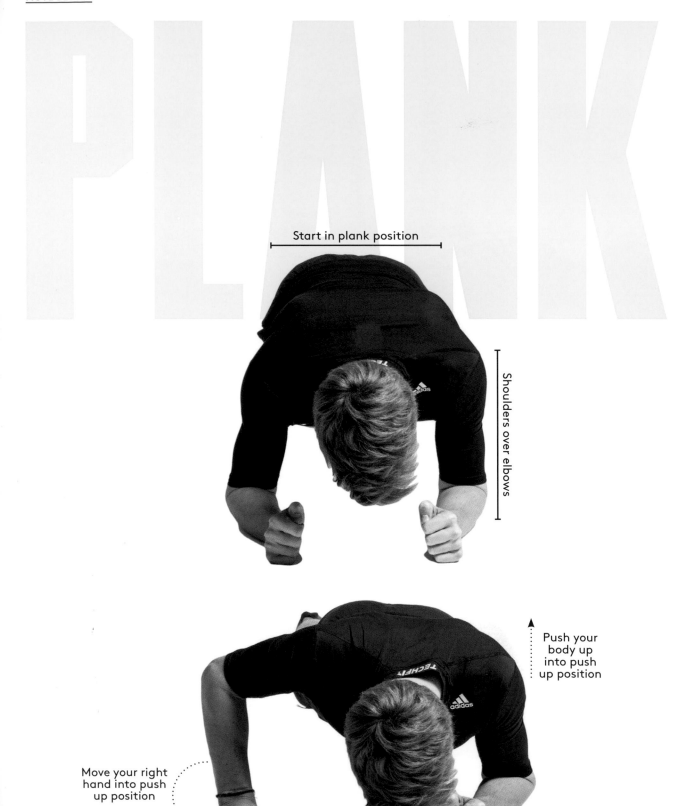

Start in plank position

Shoulders over elbows

Push your body up into push up position

Move your right hand into push up position

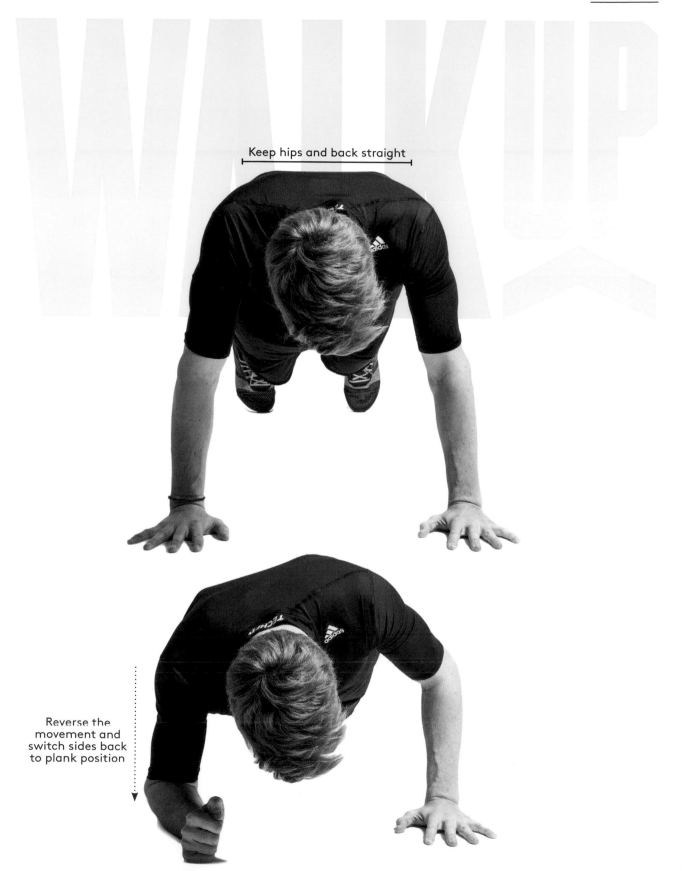

Keep hips and back straight

Reverse the movement and switch sides back to plank position

ADVANCED
HOME PLAN

DAY 1 - COMPLETE 10 MIN WARM-UP FIRST**	REPS	SETS	REST
1A ECCENTRIC SINGLE LEG BOX SQUATS	5 each leg	3	
1B BURPEES	20	3	1 min
2A ECCENTRIC STEP UPS	5 each leg	3	
2B BULGARIAN SPLIT SQUATS	10 each leg	3	1 min
3A ECCENTRIC DRAG HAMSTRING CURL	15	4	1 min
3B KETTLE BELL SWINGS OR GLUTE BRIDGE MARCH	20	4	
4A HOLLOW HOLD	30 sec	3	
4B JIU JITSU WALK THROUGHS	10 each side	3	1 min
5A V UPS	20	3	
5B BICYCLE CRUNCHES	20	3	1 min

DAY 2 - UPPER - COMPLETE 10 MIN WARM-UP FIRST**	REPS	SETS	REST
1A PULL UPS	10 (failure*)	3	
1B ECCENTRIC TRICEP PUSH UPS	12	3	1 min
2A PLANCHE PUSH UP	10	3	
2B FROG HOLD	30 sec	3	1 min
3A HANDSTAND WALL WALKS	5	4	1 min
4A SQUAT THRUSTS	20	3	
4B DIPS	20	3	1 min

* Failure is when you can no longer complete a repetition with good technique, as your muscles have fatigued.

** See page 159

In this the advanced plan we are upping the ante, not only is it 5 sessions a week but we are particularly concentrating on the ECCENTRIC[†] phase of an exercise. The eccentric phases refers to the lowering phase of a movement which is involved with deceleration; it is also when the muscle and connective tissues are under most amount of stress. This results in stronger muscles, stronger joints and thus less chance of injury. For example, the eccentric phase of a squat is the downward phase where your hips move closer to the floor.

DAY 3 - COMPLETE 10 MIN WARM-UP FIRST**

LUNGE 'N' JOG 30 MIN	2 mins of walking lunges followed by 2 mins jogging – 30 mins
CHIN UPS	See how many sets you can complete in 5 mins of chin ups then press ups.
PRESS UPS	Keep reps of each exercise to fewer than 5.

DAY 4 - CHALLENGE - COMPLETE 10 MIN WARM-UP FIRST**

	REPS
1A BURPEES	40 then 30 then 20 then 10
1B SQUATS	40 then 30 then 20 then 10
1C SIT UPS	40 then 30 then 20 then 10
20 MIN STRETCH + MOBILITY	

DAY 5 - UPPER - COMPLETE 10 MIN WARM-UP FIRST**

	REPS	SETS	REST
1A ECCENTRIC CHIN UPS	Failure*	4	2 min
2A TRICEP EXTENSION PUSH UP	8	3	
2B MULE KICKS	20	3	1 min
3A SIT UP TO HIP BRIDGE	20	3	
3B REVERSE MOUNTAIN CLIMBERS	30	4	30 sec
4A ALTERNATING ARCHERS	12	3	
4B CRUCIFIX PLANK	Failure*	3	2 min
5A HANDSTAND WALL WALKS	5	4	1 min

[†] On all eccentric movements aim for 3-5 seconds of controlled descent to really get the most from this technique.

STEP UPS

Eyes up ▸

Chest up ▸

Core tight

Weight
in heel

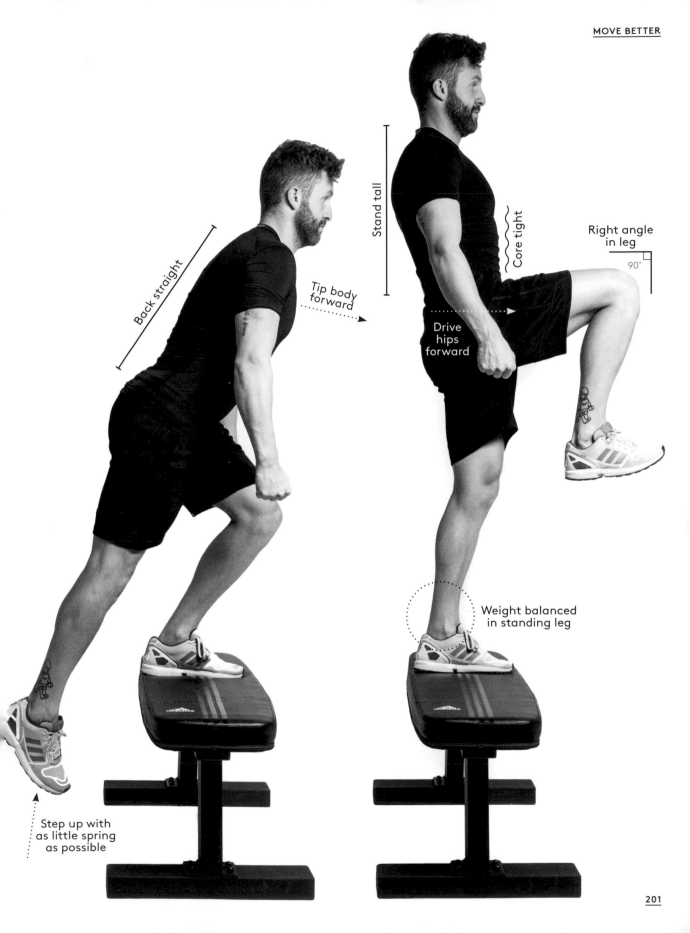

Back straight

Tip body forward

Stand tall

Core tight

Right angle in leg

90°

Drive hips forward

Weight balanced in standing leg

Step up with as little spring as possible

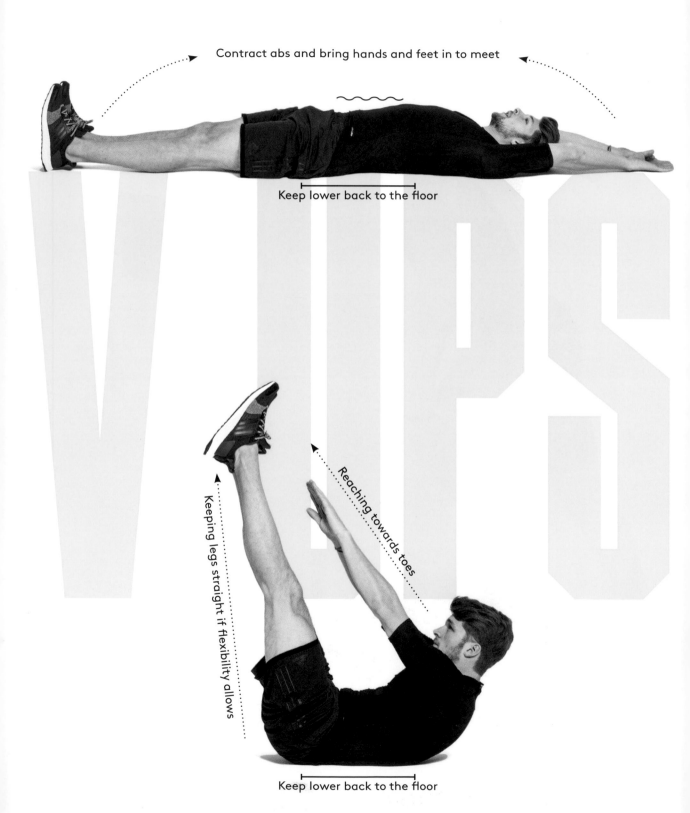

Contract abs and bring hands and feet in to meet

Keep lower back to the floor

Reaching towards toes

Keeping legs straight if flexibility allows

Keep lower back to the floor

ECCENTRIC TRICEP PUSH UPS

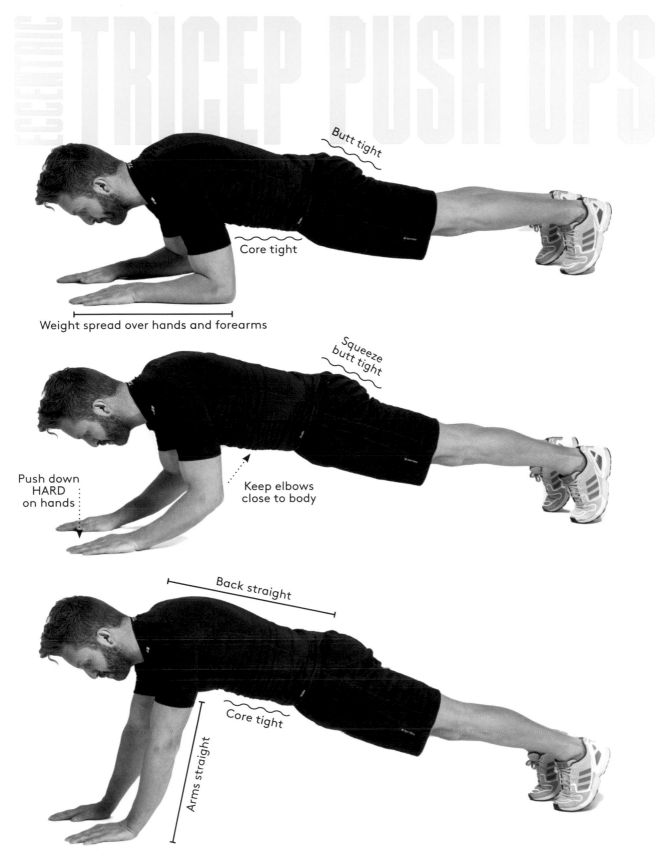

Butt tight

Core tight

Weight spread over hands and forearms

Squeeze butt tight

Push down HARD on hands

Keep elbows close to body

Back straight

Core tight

Arms straight

PLANCHE PUSH UPS

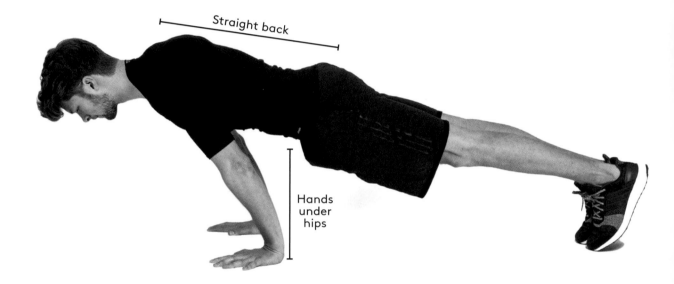

Straight back

Hands under hips

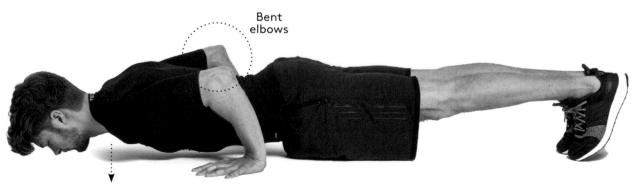

Bent elbows

Chest towards the floor

FROG

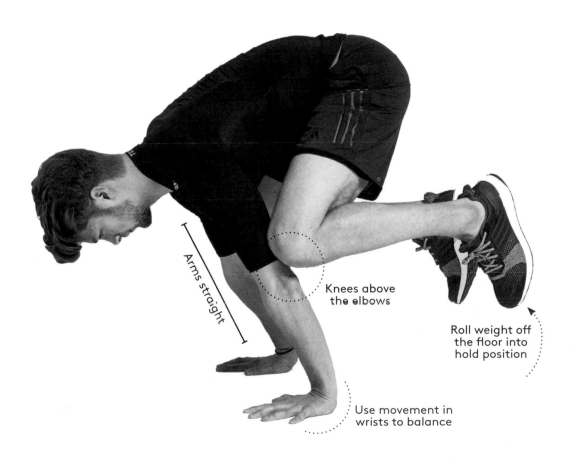

Arms straight

Knees above the elbows

Roll weight off the floor into hold position

Use movement in wrists to balance

MULE KICKS

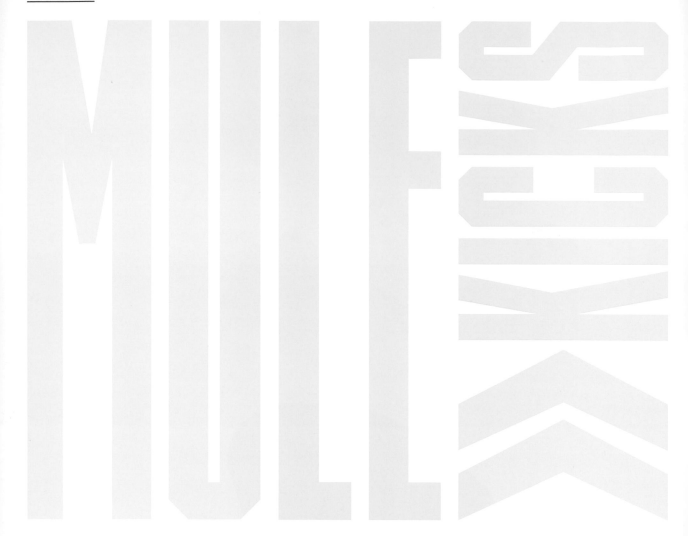

Head down

Weight over shoulders

Tuck position

Light on the feet

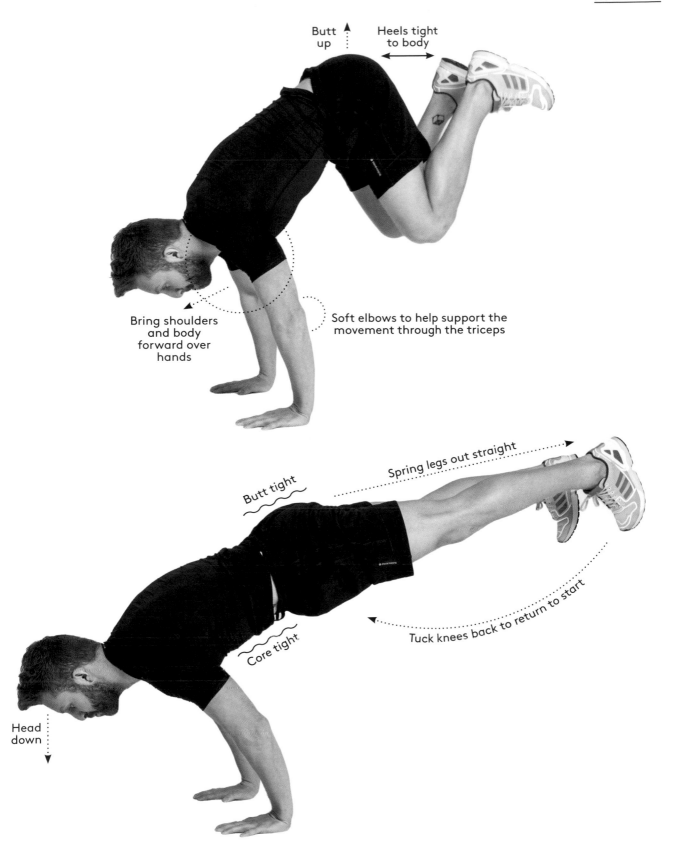

Butt
up

Heels tight
to body

Bring shoulders
and body
forward over
hands

Soft elbows to help support the
movement through the triceps

Butt tight

Spring legs out straight

Core tight

Tuck knees back to return to start

Head
down

SIT UP TO HIP BRIDGE

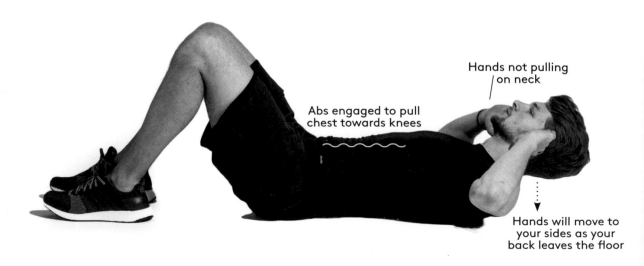

Hands not pulling on neck

Abs engaged to pull chest towards knees

Hands will move to your sides as your back leaves the floor

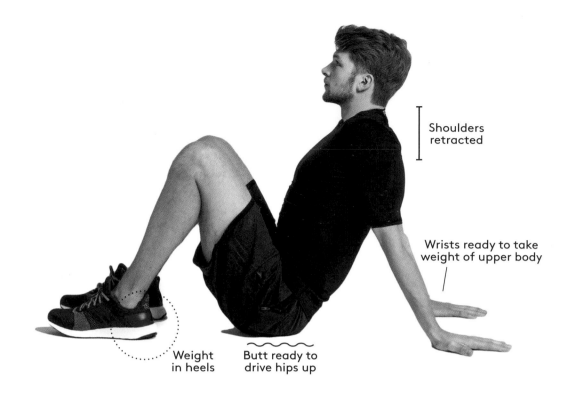

Shoulders
retracted

Wrists ready to take
weight of upper body

Weight
in heels

Butt ready to
drive hips up

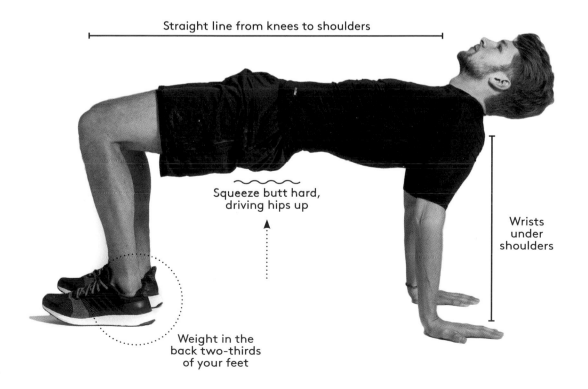

Straight line from knees to shoulders

Squeeze butt hard,
driving hips up

Wrists
under
shoulders

Weight in the
back two-thirds
of your feet

ARCHERS

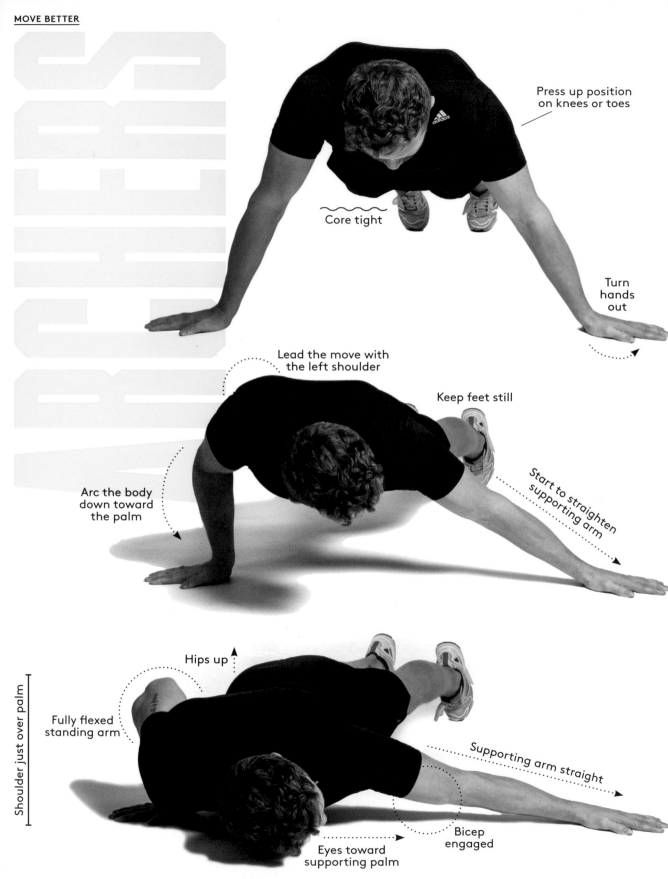

Press up position on knees or toes

Core tight

Turn hands out

Lead the move with the left shoulder

Keep feet still

Arc the body down toward the palm

Start to straighten supporting arm

Shoulder just over palm

Hips up

Fully flexed standing arm

Supporting arm straight

Eyes toward supporting palm

Bicep engaged

210

CRUCIFIX PLANK

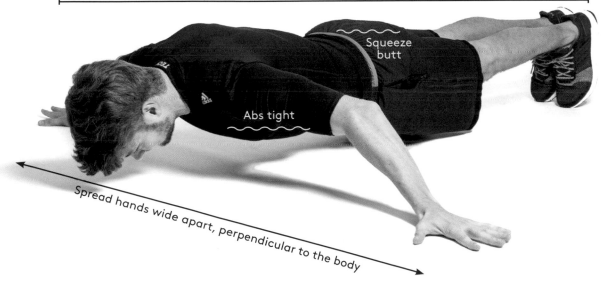

Body straight from head to heels

Squeeze butt

Abs tight

Spread hands wide apart, perpendicular to the body

GYM PLAN: 3 DAYS (BEGINNER)

Everybody will have different goals with these plans, from just getting moving more to building as much muscle as possible. With this comes certain changes and variations so we haven't written your rep ranges on the beginner plan. The most important thing is that we build good movement patterns which you can reinforce and improve.

Tempo 2-0-2-0

This may be the first time you have ever seen a tempo key but it's really simple once you know how to read it. The four numbers gauge the speed of your rep. This example means 2 seconds down (in a squat for instance), 0 break at the bottom, 2 seconds up, no break at the top. When you see an X in the tempo, this means explode (i.e. quicker than 0!).

DAY 1 - PUSH	SETS	TEMPO/NOTES
5 MIN FULL BODY DYNAMIC WARM-UP		Pulse raising movements such as body weight squats, lunges, arm swings or a gradual walk
1A SQUATS	3	2-0-2-0
2A CHEST PRESS	3	2-0-2-0
3A LUNGES	3	2-0-2-0
4A SHOULDER PRESS	3	2-0-2-0
5A STEP UPS	2	2-0-1-0
6A TRICEP PUSH DOWN TRICEP DIPS	2	2-0-1-0
UPRIGHT BIKE LV 6	1	5-15 min steady pace

DAY 2 - PULL	SETS	TEMPO/NOTES
5 MIN FULL BODY DYNAMIC WARM-UP		Pulse raising movements such as body weight squats, lunges, arm swings or a gradual walk
1A DEAD LIFTS	3	2-0-2-0
2A PULL UPS (ASSISTED)	3	2-0-2-0
3A DEAD ROW	3	2-0-2-0
4A LEG CURL	3	2-0-1-0
5A FIT BALL DRAG CURL	3	2-0-1-0
6A BARBELL CURL	2	2-0-1-0
ROWING MACHINE RESISTANCE 6	1	5-15 min steady pace

DAY 3 - FULL BODY	SETS	TEMPO/NOTES
5 MIN FULL BODY DYNAMIC WARM-UP		Pulse raising movements such as body weight squats, lunges, arm swings or a gradual walk
1A TREADMILL HIIT	6-10	20 sec 100% effort, 40 sec static recovery
1B WEIGHTED AB CRUNCH + STAR JUMPS	3	Complete both exercises before having a 45 sec break
1C LEG RAISES + HILL CLIMBERS	3	Complete both exercises before having a 45 sec break
1D WOOD CHOPS + FROG SIT UPS	3	Complete both exercises before having a 45 sec break
1E CLEAN AND PRESS + DEAD ROW	2	Complete both exercises before having a 45 sec break
1F PRESS UPS + PULL UPS	2	Complete both exercises before having a 45 sec break
1G LOWER BACK EXTENSION/DORSAL RAISE	2	Complete both exercises before having a 45 sec break

GYM PLAN: 4 DAYS (INTERMEDIATE)

The 4 day protocol is our intermediate plan, beginners are more than welcome to get stuck in on this plan too but it's quite a big jump going from no activity to 4 days so bear that in mind.

DAY 1 - FULL BODY PUSH	REPS	REST	SETS	TEMPO/NOTES
5 MIN FULL BODY DYNAMIC WARM-UP				Pulse raising movements such as body weight squats, lunges, arm swings or a gradual walk
1A SQUATS	10	1-2 min	3	3-0-1-0
2A DUMBBELL WALKING LUNGES	20 steps	1 min	3	3-0-1-0
3A FLAT DUMBBELL PRESS	10		3	3-0-1-0
3B FLAT DUMBBELL FLYS	12	1 min	3	3-0-3-0
4A DUMBBELL SHOULDER PRESS	10		3	3-0-2-0
4B TRICEP PUSH DOWN	12	1 min	3	3-0-3-0
5A HIP DRIVES	15	1 min	3	2-0-1-1

DAY 2 - FULL BODY PULL	REPS	REST	SETS	TEMPO/NOTES
5 MIN FULL BODY DYNAMIC WARM-UP				Pulse raising movements such as body weight squats, lunges, arm swings or a gradual walk
1A STIFF LEG DEAD LIFT	15	1 min	4	3-0-3-1
2A HEAVY KETTLEBELL SWING	20	1 min	3	
3A PULL UPS	10 (failure*)	1 min	4	3-0-1-0
4A DEAD ROW	10		3	3-0-2-1
4B FIT BALL HAMSTRING PULL IN	12	1 min	3	3-0-3-0
5A BARBELL CURLS	12		3	3-0-3-0
5B FACE PULLS	15	1 min	3	3-0-2-1

* Failure is when you can no longer complete a repetition with good technique, as your muscles have fatigued.

DAY 3 - FULL BODY PUSH	REPS	REST	SETS	TEMPO/NOTES
5 MIN FULL BODY DYNAMIC WARM-UP				Pulse raising movements such as body weight squats, lunges, arm swings or a gradual walk
1A LEG PRESS	15	1 min	4	3-0-2-0
2A WEIGHTED HIGH STEP UP	10 each leg	1 min	3	2-0-X-1
3A MILITARY PRESS	12	1 min	3	3-0-1-0
4A INCLINE DUMBBELL PRESS	12		3	3-0-2-0
4B SKULL CRUSHERS	10	1 min	3	3-0-2-1
5A LEG EXTENSION	12		3	3-0-3-0
5B HIP DRIVES	8-10	1 min	3	2-0-1-0

DAY 4 - FULL BODY PULL	REPS	REST	SETS	TEMPO/NOTES
5 MIN FULL BODY DYNAMIC WARM-UP				Pulse raising movements such as body weight squats, lunges, arm swings or a gradual walk
1A DEAD LIFT	8-10	1-2 min	4	3-1-2-1
2A LAYING LEG CURL	12	1 min	3	3-0-2-0
3A CLOSE GRIP CHIN UPS	10 (failure*)	1 min	3	2-0-1-0
4A SINGLE ARM ROW	8 each arm		3	3-0-2-0
4B CABLE CURL	15	1 min	3	3-0-3-0
5A REAR DELT RAISE	15		3	2-0-2-0
5B HAMMER CURL	8 each arm	1 min	3	2-0-2-0

GYM PLAN: 5 DAYS (ADVANCED)

This advanced plan is not for the faint hearted and starts to split your training into different body parts meaning each muscle group gets more focus in a single session (remember progressive overload). Keep noting down your reps and weights so you can track your progress!

If you are more experienced with your training you may choose to periodise your plan for example:

- week 1-2:   6 reps (strength)
- week 2-3:   10-12 reps (hypertrophy)
- weeks 3-4: 15-20 reps (volume)

You may also choose to do your cardio on separate sessions using steady state or suggested GYM HIIT protocols. Good Luck!

DAY 1 - CHEST + TRICEPS	REPS	REST	SETS	TEMPO/NOTES
5 MIN DYNAMIC WARM-UP				
1A FLAT BENCH PRESS	8-10	1 min	4	3-0-2-0
2A INCLINE BENCH	12	1 min	4	3-0-2-0
3A WEIGHTED DIPS	8	1 min	3	3-0-2-0
4A CABLE FLYS	12		3	3-0-2-0
4B PRESS UPS	Failure*	45 sec	3	3-0-1-0
5A PUSH DOWN	12		3	3-0-2-0
5B TRICEP PUSH UP	Failure*	45 sec	3	3-0-1-0
INCLINE WALK 10'			1	10 min fast walking pace

DAY 2 - LEGS	REPS	REST	SETS	TEMPO/NOTES
5 MIN DYNAMIC WARM-UP				
1A SQUATS	6	2-3 min	3	3-0-X-0
2A WALKING LUNGES	10 each leg	1 min	3	3-0-2-0
3A HIP DRIVES	15		3	3-0-2-0
3B WEIGHTED STEP UPS	6 each leg	90 sec	3	2-1-2-1
4A LEG EXTENSION	12	1 min	3	2-0-2-0
5A HAMSTRING CURL	12	1 min	3	2-0-2-0
UPRIGHT BIKE			1	10 min moderate speed lv 8-14

* Failure is when you can no longer complete a repetition
  with good technique, as your muscles have fatigued.

DAY 3 - BACK + BICEPS	REPS	REST	SETS	TEMPO/NOTES
5 MIN DYNAMIC WARM-UP				
1A DEAD LIFTS	5	3-5 min	5	2-1-X-0
2A PULL UPS	10 (failure*)		4	3-0-X-0
3A T BAR ROWS	10		3	3-0-2-0
3B FACE PULLS	15	1 min	3	3-0-2-1
4A SINGLE ARM ROW	8-10 each side		3	3-0-2-0
4B LYING DUMBBELL CURL	10	1 min	3	3-0-2-1
5A BARBELL CURL	15	1 min	3	3-0-1-1
ROWING MACHINE			1	2000m steady state row resistance 6-9

DAY 4 - SHOULDERS + CORE	REPS	REST	SETS	TEMPO/NOTES
1A MILITARY PRESS	6	1-2 min	4	2-0-2-0
2A DUMBBELL SEATED PRESS	12	1 min	3	3-0-2-0
3A FARMERS WALKS	20 steps	1 min	3	
4A REAR DELT RAISES	10		3	2-0-2-0
4B SIDE RAISES	15	1 min	3	2-0-2-0
5A PLANCHE PUSH UPS	Failure*	1 min	3	2-0-2-0
AB CIRCUIT:			3	
20 HANGING LEG RAISE				
20 WEIGHTED CRUNCH				
20 SLOW ROTATIONS				
20 V UPS				

DAY 5 - LEGS	REPS	REST	SETS	TEMPO/NOTES
5 MIN DYNAMIC WARM-UP				3-0-3-0
1A STIFF LEG DEAD LIFTS	15	1 min	4	3-0-3-0
2A LEG PRESS	8	1-2 min	4	3-0-2-0
3A HIP DRIVES	10	1 min	3	3-0-2-1
4A GOBLET SQUATS	15		3	3-0-3-0
4B LEG CURL	10	1 min	3	3-0-2-0
5A FITBALL DRAG IN	15	1 min	3	3-0-3-0
X-TRAINER			1	10 min steady state lv 8-14

HOME HIGH INTENSITY PLAN
Every circuit is to be completed from the first to last exercise with no break inbetween, followed by a 90 second recovery before completing another set.

HIIT 1 - BEGINNER	REPS	SETS	NOTES
5-10 MIN WARM-UP			
MOUNTAIN CLIMBERS	20 sec sprint	2	
PRESS UPS	15	2	Optional: on knees
JUMP SQUATS	15	2	
SQUAT THRUSTS	15	2	
PLANK	30 sec	2	
RECOVERY	90 sec		

HIIT 2 - INTERMEDIATE	REPS	SETS	NOTES
5-10 MIN WARM-UP			
BURPEES	15	3	
STAR JUMPS	30	3	
PLYO LUNGES	15 each leg	3	
PLANK THRUSTS	15	3	
PRESS UP + OPEN	15 each way	3	
V-SITS	15	3	
RECOVERY	90 sec		

HIIT 3 - ADVANCE INVERSE LADDERS			NOTES
5-10 MINS WARM-UP			
BURPEES	10		1 rep each set
SQUAT JUMPS	10		1 rep each set
PRESS UPS	10		1 rep each set
V-SITS	10		1 rep each set
RECOVERY	90 sec		

This is what we call inverse ladders. You do 10 reps of each of the four exercises then with little to no break go back to the start and do 9, then 8, then 7 and so on. You finish once you're down to a single rep of each exercise. This is only to be completed once through.

GYM HIGH INTENSITY PLAN

These are high intensity circuits which require gym equipment.

HIIT 1 - BEGINNER: X-TRAINER 15 MIN	TIME	LEVEL	NOTES
5-10 MIN WARM-UP			
100% EFFORT SPRINT	30 sec	15	Level is specific to you but you don't want to feel that you can't keep up with your legs
RECOVERY	60 sec	5	

HIIT 2 - INTERMEDIATE: ROWER SPRINTS 10-15 MIN	TIME	NOTES
5-10 MIN WARM-UP		
100% EFFORT SPRINT	200m	Repeat for 10-15 min
RECOVERY PACE 30%	60 sec	

HIIT 3 - ADVANCED: DEADMILL* SPRINTS 10 MIN	TIME	SETS
5-10 MIN WARM-UP		
100% PUSH SPRINTS	20 sec	10
STOP FOR RECOVERY	40 sec	10

*Treadmill does not get turned on as you use the motor as resistance. Not for the faint hearted!

CONCLUSION

We hope that you enjoyed our book and it has helped you, whether that be in terms of nutrition, exercise or just knowing that it's OK to be who you want to be.

Please feel free to share your thoughts, experiences and progressions with us via our social platforms using the hashtag #TLM. We always love to hear from you.

 @TheLeanMachines TheLeanMachines TheLeanMachines @theleanmachinesofficial

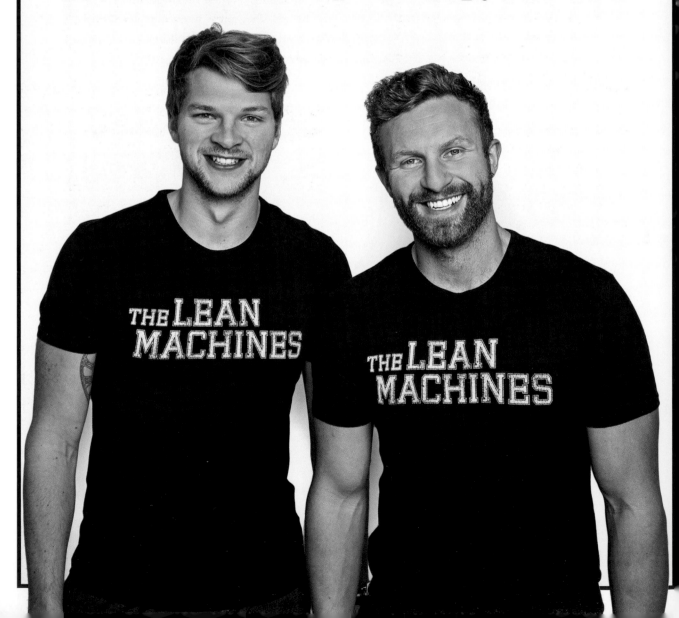

ACKNOWLEDGEMENTS

We want to take a moment to say a few thank yous, starting with our partners Rosie and Carly for putting up with the long nights, our constant read throughs and for always supporting us in everything we do.

Our mindset coach Stephen Aish was one of the first people who opened our eyes to the true power of the mind and living your life in the present. The journey we've been on and the people we've become with his help is very AWESOME.

We had a huge leg up in our careers thanks to our good friend and gym manager Shaun Cable, we have to say a huge thank you to you Shaun. You were the first person who gave us a chance, believed in us and gave us a platform in the fitness industry by giving us our first job and allowing us to train clients within the gym environment.

Maddie & Charlotte (manager & producer at Gleam). These two are just legendary at keeping everything together. They support our passion and more importantly understand it. Without these two The Lean Machines would be pure chaos! Also a huge thank you to Natalie who is no longer part of the team but was a massive part of The Lean Machines up until last year.

A huge thank you to Rich Harris for helping us to create some truly incredible recipes that look great and taste even better, and to Laura Herring for all your help.

To Headline the publishers who 'get' The Lean Machines and our message, passion and beliefs. They came to us, supported and developed this beautiful creation, and worked alongside us every step of the way.

The guys at Well Made Studio designed all the graphics and pretty much brought our book to life, they're an incredibly talented group of people and so easy to work with.

But MOST IMPORTANTLY to YOU the subscribers and readers: Thank you to every single one of you who have supported our journey, whether you've been watching since that first most awkward and uncomfortable video or if this book was our first meeting, your support means the world so thank you.